THE EXPECTANT FATHER

by

STEVEN JEFFREY BERGER

dp
DISTINCTIVE PUBLISHING CORP.

The Expectant Father
By Steven Jeffrey Berger

Published by Distinctive Publishing Corp.
P. O. Box 17868
Plantation, FL 33318-7868
Printed in the United States of America

ISBN: 0-942963-40-7
Library of Congress No.: 93-36432
Price: $7.95

Library of Congress Cataloging-in-Publication Data

Berger, Steven Jeffrey, 1961-
The expectant father / by Steven Jeffrey Berger.
p. cm.
ISBN 0-942963-40-7 (tradesoft) : 7.95
1. Fathers—Humor. 2. Pregnancy—Humor. 3. Childbirth—Humor.
I. Title.
HQ756.B46 1993 93-36432
306.874'2—dc20 CIP

With love and gratitude for my wife, Anita.

- 1 -

My day had begun as any other typical Monday morning. Like countless others everywhere, I was doing my best to shake off the weekend's reprieve and preparing myself to face another week at the office. I showered, shaved, got dressed, chained up the dog in the garage, and headed for work.

Now, in order to convey the truest intent of this book, it will be necessary from time to time to depart from the basic story line (if indeed there ever is one) and give specific detail to certain references made. Already there are two such instances: chaining up the dog in the garage and what I do to earn a living.

I am very familiar with the expression, "Dog is man's best friend." I have also no doubt that in the majority of households in which a canine has residence, the average Fido, Spot and Rover is well adjusted to the average Tom, Dick and Harry. With respect to my own case, however, the proper adjustment has never quite taken place.

The dog in my household is named Rastus. He is a purebred miniature dachshund (a.k.a. "the weiner dog") of whom I became proud owner as a result of my marriage, some fourteen months earlier. Actually, my wife had inherited Rastus, while he was still a puppy, from her mother, who had passed away several years prior to that.

I always found it downright fascinating that my deceased mother-in-law, whom I never really had the chance to know, had faced death with very little personal want beyond owning a dachshund dog. As the fulfillment of a dying request, more or less, she had been presented with Rastus as a Christmas present by her husband, my wife's father. The dog lived with its original owner for approximately six months, during which time it was given complete charge of the house.

Not surprisingly, my father-in-law, who is primarily revered for his intelligence and overall good business sense, decided upon his wife's passing to seek a new residence for Rastus. As a matter of course, my wife and her first husband became the dog's adoptive parents. Although their marriage failed, the dog thrived. And as both fate and my wife would have it, upon my saying "I Do," I became the second stepfather to *Rastus, the Dachshund Dog*.

As for my desire to openly welcome Rastus into my life, trust me, it was sincere. But try as I might to afford the dog the same liberties it had enjoyed living with its previous owners, what I found was that the four-legged creature could simply not be trusted in the house alone, be it for eight hours or eight minutes. And I'm not just talking about your standard *steaming surprise* left on the living room carpet. I'm talking about chewed up rugs, chewed up clothes, chewed up furniture, and then your standard steaming surprise left on the living room carpet. In spite of it all, however, insisting that his presence be removed was completely out of the question.

It was no secret that, for my wife, the dog represented a very strong emotional tie to her deceased mother. It was also understood that where he went, she would follow. Considering that I had more than just a glimpse of the dog's character prior to getting married, I couldn't quite justify his existence as a legitimate grounds for divorce. In short, I was stuck with him.

There was always room for compromise, however. And the compromise here was the agreement that during any absence from our home, Rastus would be confined to the garage. To be specific, he was to be kept on a twelve-foot leash—limiting, yes, but keep in mind that the dog only stood six inches high.

Now before the reader is compelled to report me to the A.S.P.C.A., it should be noted that what the dog was actually chained to was a custom built dog house complete with a heater, food, water, blankets, and various chew toys—a veritable puppy paradise, or so it seemed to me. Rastus, however, did not share this belief, and in spite of his being given all the comforts of home, he never willingly accepted his daily incarceration within the garage. Unfortunately for me—because my wife typically left the house before I did—convincing the dog that this was his particular lot in life normally fell under my domain of responsibility.

At first my approach to getting the dog into the garage had been fairly straightforward. It consisted simply of confronting the animal while it slept and extracting its ten-pound body from under the covers where it was burrowed. Given my definite advantage of about a hundred and seventy pounds, this seemed to be a sound approach. However, given the dog's reaction of attempting to inject its teeth into both my hands, it was an approach that I had utilized for all of about two days. Hence came plan "B."

Plan "B" was actually more of a concentrated campaign than any one particular approach. The whole point was to get the dog out of bed on its own accord, enabling me to scoop him up without causing harm to myself in the process. If it required a bit of deception on my part, so be it.

There was no denying that Rastus had proven to be the victor in hand-to-hand combat. When it came to the art of psychological warfare, however, he was really no match at all. I would keep him guessing by varying my methods, which, to name a few, included: standing on the front porch pretending to be a door-to-door salesman, jingling a leash in the guise that we were going for a walk, and waving a bag of catnip in the air to simulate the presence of the dog's natural enemy. They were all successful means of tricking Rastus out of bed. My really big gun, however, was appealing to the dog's sense of food.

For anyone unfamiliar with the innate habits of dachshunds—what you must realize is that they possess an insatiable appetite and will do virtually anything when there is a prospect of receiving food. Even after being fed, the dachshund will still act as if it hasn't eaten in a week. I must confess that on an occasion or two, I have used this aspect of the dog's nature for my own misguided pleasure. One incident in particular related to a dinner given by my wife and me for our two closest friends, Chris and Jenny Graham.

As was customary in our gatherings with the Grahams, the conversation often included reminiscent childhood stories. On this specific night, my wife had told the very sad, albeit twistedly amusing tale, of her childhood pet, Beave, a guinea pig. Apparently Beave had been given too much food and, not knowing when to stop eating, had literally exploded from over consumption.

I've always considered myself a man of compassion and gentle persuasion. Listening to the story of Beave's unfortunate demise, however—while Rastus incessantly *humped* my foot under the table—I was beginning to entertain some very unscrupulous ideas. Later that night I volunteered to do the dishes, knowing full well that Rastus would be dancing around my feet every moment, dreaming of having something fall into his grasp.

From this particular dinner, there had been an unusual amount of leftovers—including nearly four full servings of a delicious, but extremely rich, chocolate mousse. The story of Beave's over indulgence was running rampant in my mind, and as I tripped over Rastus while reaching for a towel, I just sort of—all at once—went snap.

I started with the salad, then the French bread, then the remnants of baked potatoes, then the asparagus with Hollandaise sauce, and finally the steak scraps. All of it was piled high into the shiny tin bowl. Rastus chomped furiously at the mound of heaven before him, completely oblivious to the evil intent behind his good fortune.

I was amazed that within a moment, he had not only finished, but was asking for more. I beheld the chocolate mousse, fully aware that this was not an item on the animal's recommended diet. Nevertheless, he definitely seemed to want it.

One at a time, I tipped the long stemmed dessert glasses, whipped cream and all, into the dog's dish. After two servings, not to mention everything else he had consumed, Rastus showed absolutely no sign of slowing down. I emptied the third glass and found myself cheering, "Come on Beave, go pop for Daddy." Just as I had begun to administer the fourth and largest serving, my wife appeared.

She had surmised my plan instantly, and with a move that Robin Hood would have envied, swiftly swung down to rescue Rastus from harm. Knowing that I was surely about to be judged for my crime, all I could think to say on my own behalf was, "Boy, Honey, he sure was hungry."

The defense unheard, I was sentenced to a night on the couch. Needless to say, my side of the bed was kept warm that night by Rastus. Although I never did witness any ill effect from my misconduct toward the dog, my wife swears that, "He slept a bit uneasy that evening." But enough of my tales of "Rastus the Dachshund Dog." I turn back to the particular morning in question.

I had left the house that day at about 8:15 a.m. Ignoring the dog's protest, I climbed into my car and was soon sputtering my way among the ranks of rush hour commuters.

I must admit that, as a child, I hadn't given a lot of thought to what I'd do when I grew up. It wasn't that I lacked ambition. It was simply a case of lacking direction, which led me to become embedded in a career that I could in no way have foreseen.

I worked as a sales manager for a substantially sized insurance company. The truth was that in the beginning, I had taken a job for the sole purpose of providing immediate income. The irony was that in spite of the complete lack of regard that I held for my particular profession, I kept getting promoted. (Perhaps this very lack of regard was a prerequisite for advancement; I don't know.) At any rate, devoid of any conscious attempt, I somehow went from being an individual with just a job, to being an individual with a budding career.

In all candor, regardless of whatever emotional conflict I may have felt toward my job, the tangible benefits were indisputably rewarding. Beyond the perks of a company car and expense account, the pay itself was downright tantalizing. These were the decisive pros that compelled me to continue to show up for work on a daily basis. The downside, however, was that the more I seemed to make, the more I seemed to spend. What I ate, how I dressed, the European sports sedan in the garage—this was all a product of my increasingly upward financial status.

There was something else that I was beginning to notice in affiliation with my professional success—the more stable I became in my career, the more turbulent things seemed to be in my personal life.

Over the previous fourteen months alone, I had not only become a married man, but had purchased a home as well. These were radical events that increasingly seemed to please the people who wrote my paycheck every two weeks. Nevertheless, they were changes that made me wonder if a little consistency might not be so bad for a while.

But I was at that caught-between-age of transition—twenty-seven. I was too old to shirk responsibility under the claim of adolescence, yet too young to say with any conviction that I knew what I wanted for the rest of my life. For now, it seemed that the only appropriate thing to do was to push on and assume that eventually it would all make perfect sense. And so I did, indeed, push on.

By 9:00 a.m., I was behind my desk reviewing the to do list I had left the Friday afternoon before. It was going to be a hectic day. But provided that I remained focused, I saw no reason for my not being able to complete the tasks before me. I was about to begin with the morning mail when the phone rang.

Monday mornings are always full of interruptions. It never fails to amaze me how the week always starts on such a crisis basis. Reaching for the phone, I was prepared to "drop everything" and race off to a meeting of the "utmost importance." Of course such meetings were usually never very important at all, and I often wondered if there was just some unknown quota to fill. It was a pleasant surprise, however, to find that it was actually my wife's voice on the other end of the line.

"Hi, Honey, what's up?"

From the silence that ensued, my guess was that this was not going to be one of those "just calling to say that I love you and to see what you wanted for dinner" type of phone calls. On the contrary, my instinct compelled me to brace myself for whatever shocking news that I was about to receive.

I inquired again: "What's the matter? Is everything okay?"

There was no hesitation this time before my wife's response. Clearly, concisely, and in a very matter of fact tone of voice, she said two words that left me absolutely stunned: "I'm pregnant."

I can't say with any degree of accuracy how long it was that I just sat there holding the receiver in the air. All I know is that it was a faint voice repeating my name over and over again that served as the proverbial smelling salts to help me regain my composure.

"Steven? Steven? Are you there?"

I was there all right—somewhat dazed and more than just a bit confused, but definitely there.

My mind was racing. I felt an urgency to establish the facts behind the big story that had just made the front page of my life.

"Why didn't you say anything? You should have told me if you thought you were pregnant."

"Well, I didn't want to say anything until I knew for sure. Now that I know, I'm telling you!"

This was true; she was certainly telling me.

"Well, how far along are you?"

"The doctor thinks about two months. But I've got to go back in a few weeks for some additional tests to get a better idea. Look, why don't you just come home so we can talk about it? I'd much rather play the game of twenty questions face to face than over the phone."

My wife was right. If ever there was a legitimate cause to "drop everything" and deal with the issue at hand, this was it. We concluded our conversation and I immediately proceeded to place a call to my boss.

Upon informing him of my impending parenthood, the response I received was one of wholehearted congratulations. As for taking the remainder of the day off, it was his suggestion that I take the next several days off as well, "Just to sort of let it all sink in." He then went on to offer his unsolicited opinion of, “We gotcha now, kid.”

I didn’t at all agree with the closing comment my boss had made. Still, I shuddered at the very thought of any validity it may have contained. Either way, as I left my office for the journey back home, I couldn’t help muttering my own profound observation: “So much for a little consistency for a while.”

- 2 -

It was Franklin Delano Roosevelt, thirty-third President of the United States, who, during one of the darkest times in the nation's history, immortalized the words: *"We have nothing to fear, except fear itself."*

Was it just a maneuver — a politician's ploy — of utilizing a clever cliché to merely distract the people's attention from the dramatically disheartening events taking place? Or had FDR and his speech writers truly felt that they were presenting the masses with a household cure for the emotionally crippling disease of anxiety?

"Nothing to fear but fear itself." I had always believed in those words. And yet, as I drove back home that morning repeating them over and over again, I was absolutely petrified of what I imagined the future might hold. I found myself recalling the simpler days of my youth.

It was intriguing how vivid it all seemed. I remembered being seven years old and playing race car driver behind the wheel of my parents' car. And then I was thirteen and rounding the bases after hitting the game-winning homer. The next stop was several years later, visiting a first love and having the great fortune of leaving behind my virginity.

With every mile that the odometer ticked off, it seemed that another year of my life flashed by. And then suddenly, the clock froze and settled on a late August morning in the not-too-distant past—my wedding day.

The wedding chapel of the Bally's Hotel in Reno, Nevada, was a room that easily accommodated seventy-five people. For the particular ceremony in which I was involved, however, the attendance was limited to myself, my wife-to-be, and a minister named "Rick," who wore a tie tack that proclaimed: "Reno,

The Biggest Little City In The World."

Technically speaking, we had eloped. The manner in which we became husband and wife, however, was not the result of two romantically lost, impetuous souls. It was true that we shared an immense love for each other. But our decision to partake in a *quickie* marriage was based solely on necessity. Allow me to expound on that point.

During the two-and-a-half-year courting period that had preceded, my wife and I did not enjoy what one might call a *stable* relationship. Quite the contrary. It would be far more accurate to describe our romance as *highly volatile*, much like a flask of nitroglycerin released from a great height and allowed to plummet freely to the ground. It wasn't a question of "if" there would be an explosion—only a question of "how large?"

The problem was that in spite of being in love with each other, we didn't like each other much. It wasn't anyone's fault. It was simply the case that aside from our domineering personalities, we really didn't have a whole lot in common. To make matters worse, neither of us was particularly skilled at showing any respect for the other's difference of opinion. As a result, we became highly proficient at the art of breaking up.

On the flip side, however, as often as we ended our relationship, there were just as many times in which we found the means to reinstate it. It was a phenomenon that seemed to absolutely baffle those who knew us, but we were extremely good at it.

Still, after two years of playing break-up/make-up, there was no question that it was time to reach a conclusion about what to do with each other. It was for that reason that we agreed to move in together, allowing ourselves six months to decide whether we should get married or part ways, once and for all.

And so it was that we rented a small, albeit quaint, house by the lake. We hung pictures, placed our names on the mailbox, and selected a permanent corner in the kitchen for Rastus' dish. In short, we made the little house our home.

In retrospect, I must admit that I had no real expectation of a long-term commitment evolving from this all or nothing step taken in our relationship. In fact, the only expectation I remember having was that in six months, I would be faced with the task of seeking a new residence. With this perspective in mind, I was well prepared for the fateful day in which there would, no doubt, be tears, but also the consolation of finally moving on with our lives. (It was callous, I know, but keep in mind that I'm being honest.)

With about five weeks remaining in our arrangement, my job required me to travel for a two-week series of seminars. For the majority of my colleagues, the news of such a lengthy absence from home was a cause of great discontent. I, however, viewed it as a welcome prelude to the final separation which I believed was scheduled soon to take place. I also saw it as a tremendous opportunity to better get to know a fellow employee, whom, for the purpose of anonymity, I shall refer to as Susan.

I had known Susan for a little more than a year. Although we reported to different departments, we had worked together on a number of projects, during which we discovered that a strong sense of chemistry seemed to exist between us. I found her not only attractive, but also intelligent, charming and witty. She was well respected by her peers and was no doubt destined for a brilliant career within our organization. All and all, I guess you could say that I considered Susan to be the perfect woman.

In spite of several flirtatious encounters, I had never really given any thought to the idea of Susan and I actually going out on a date. I had, after all—for the entire time I had known her—been involved in a somewhat trying, but nevertheless loving, on again, off again, relationship. At this particular time, however, completely believing that the relationship back home was truly about to come to a close, I saw absolutely no reason for Susan and me not to go out together. Fate seemed to agree with me, for Susan readily accepted my invitation to a romantic, candlelight dinner for two.

I suppose that sitting across the table and staring longingly into Susan's eyes, I was anticipating that the heavens were about to open, offering me admittance to some higher plane of both pleasure and understanding. At last, I was standing on the other side of the fence, knee deep in a far greener pasture.

Over wine, we talked about work-related issues and shared

our views on the seminar we were attending. Things were going well, but I was compelled to get to know this person on more than just a professional level. Realizing the opportunity before me, I took a chance:

"Tell me, Susan, what are your dreams in life?"

I had asked that question with every degree of sensitivity that I possessed. I was also poised with the utmost attention to receive its response. As the answer came, however, I could feel the blades of the lush green grass beneath me begin to whither and die. So rapid and unexpected was the transformation that, within moments, I found myself standing in a veritable dust bowl.

Susan's most inner aspirations consisted of an orderly series of events, all beginning with finding a "suitable" man to marry. Once that task had been accomplished, she and her husband would occupy a somewhat modest, albeit quintessential suburban home, complete with a white picket fence. In the backyard there would be a dog, preferably a collie, and in the garage there would be a station wagon, preferably a Volvo, in which she would transport the children, all five of them, back and forth to school, Girl Scouts, and Little League functions alike. She would, of course, like to give up her job, in order to concentrate on more altruistic matters such as the P.T.A., church affiliations and other worthwhile community affairs.

I don't remember having asked for a sign of divine guidance that night, but that is precisely how I was interpreting my date with Susan to be. As she continued to expound on her version of the *ideal life*, I began to realize how limited my own life would be, due to the abundance of preconceived notions and expectations I had established for myself. I was still staring into Susan's eyes, but it was now a vacant stare. My thoughts became centered on the girl back home, who, at the moment, was some seven hundred miles away.

It was suddenly clear how foolish I had been. For more than two years, there'd been a woman in my life—a woman who, in absence, had made my heart absolutely ache. And yet, I had never been able to accept the way I felt about this woman because she was so different than what I ever imagined she should be. Regardless of how whole this person made me feel, I had been convinced that there was someone else more *suitable* for me, perhaps waiting just up ahead. Up until this night, I thought that *someone* might have been Susan. It was ironic that it took Susan to make me realize that the someone I'd been waiting for was already there, waiting for me.

Or was she?

My mind began to race with panic. What if I were to return home to only a note saying, "Goodbye, forever"? It was possible—even probable—that as I sat there with Susan, some smooth and suave character was convincing the one true love of my life what a fool she had been for wasting her time on the likes of me. Repeatedly, I had refused to give any indication beyond the want of a temporary relationship. And now that I was ready and willing to make a firm commitment, I feared it was too late.

Time was of the essence. There might still be a chance that I could salvage that which I had sought to destroy. But I had to act quickly. The immediate obstacle was Susan. As I was searching for the means to a tactful exit, our food arrived.

There were two particular thoughts that came to mind. One was to simply tell Susan the truth and hope for the best. The other was to forgo any risk of emotional complications and feign a sudden physical distress. However, possessing neither the courage for the former nor the acting ability for the latter, I decided that it would be my appropriate penance to just sit there and suffer. And suffer I did. It was bad enough that dinner seemed to last an eternity. But thanks to the waiter's insistence, Susan agreed to try the specialty of the house dessert, chocolate soufflé, promised as, "Well worth the mere thirty minutes it would take to prepare."

At last, the check arrived. The manner in which I paid the bill made it more than obvious that I was, indeed, in a hurry to vacate the premises. Susan commented that she was sorry for the additional time for her dessert. I wanted to tell her that I was the one who should be saying, "I'm sorry," and for a lot more than just a leisurely meal. But I saw the matter of the soufflé as a prime opportunity to conclude the evening.

I told her that I'd forgotten to make an extremely important phone call earlier and asked her forgiveness in returning directly to the hotel. She was very gracious about the matter and responded that there was no apology necessary.

So there I was, finally alone in my room. The sense of urgency that had dawned nearly three hours ago had not subsided. I grabbed the phone and poked furiously at the numbered pad. As the sound of varying musical notes gave way to the less melodic, monotone ring, my heart was pounding. Then it literally stopped, as I recognized the voice coming through the receiver: "Hello?'

I hadn't thought at all about what I was going to say. Whether or not the words to describe the way I felt even existed, I wasn't sure. All I knew was that at that moment, the most important thing in the world was to somehow convey the immense love that I held for this person on the other end of the line.

I won't pretend to have remembered the exact conversation. I do recall, however, that after the obligatory questions—"How are you? Hope I'm not disturbing you?"—I came right out with my proposal of marriage. I also recall, distinctly, the response with which it was met:

"Are you drunk or something?"

Now I admit that the radical change in my attitude did warrant a bit of skepticism. But it was within the realm of reality.

"Of course I'm not drunk. I'm in love with you, and I want to marry you."

"Yeah, right. That's why I'm getting calls asking if you still want to see the apartment. Why didn't you tell me you were moving out?"

"I was only thinking about moving out, assuming that things were not going to work out between us."

"And now you want to get married?"

Okay, so it did sound a little implausible, but there was no denying the thunderbolt that had struck me.

"But you have to marry me. If you don't, I'll never fall in love with anyone else. I know that because I'll never be able to stop being in love with you."

"Well, maybe, but it still sounds a little fishy, if you ask me."

It was a debate that lasted for nearly an hour—I, continuing to profess my undying love; she, continuing to stand firm on the dubiousness of my sincerity. But my persistence prevailed. Thirty-three fifty in phone charges later, I heard the magical word that made me believe I was the luckiest man alive:

"Yes."

There was only one stipulation that I was required to accept—we were to become married at the first available opportunity. Upon my inquiry of, "Why?" I was told that with all the tumult we had already endured, I would not be given the chance to change my mind. Although I took this as something of a smudge against my character, I readily conceded to the condition imposed.

The first available opportunity proved to be several weeks later, when we found ourselves on a Monday at 10:00 a.m., standing side by side before the alter of the Bally's Hotel Wedding Chapel in Reno, Nevada. There we bonded our souls and spirits together in holy matrimony, in a ceremony officiated by Minister "Rick" and his rather opulent tie tack.

Those were the facts behind our elopement. And to think, less than fourteen months later, a child was on the way.

By the time I finally arrived home, I was emotionally drained. I had witnessed a first hand version of "This is Your Life," and I wasn't quite sure how to react to the show's conclusion.

I suppose that standing there on the front steps, I looked all grown up in my pin striped suit, my briefcase in hand. The truth, however, was that I had the overwhelming desire to be thirteen again, rounding the bases on the ball field just one more time. But that was a secret I was determined not to tell.

I entered the house to find my wife standing in the hall to greet me. The expression on her face was the same as the one I was desperately fighting not to show—complete and utter fear. Without saying a word, we just stood there and held onto each other. After a few moments, we moved into the living room to discuss the situation at hand.

We were a relatively young couple. My wife had recently returned to college to pursue her undergraduate degree. Still, judged against the hardships of others, we were certainly capable—both financially and emotionally—to take on the responsibility of a child. It was mainly the timing of it all that seemed to have caught us so incredibly off guard.

From the onset of our marriage, we had each spoken favorably about having children. But it was always in the hypothetical context of *somewhere* in the future. I, as did my wife, had always interpreted that to mean a time years and years away. That morning, however, we came to the shocking realization that the term somewhere had been drastically reduced to the approximate seven months remaining, in which we would have to prepare to become Mommy and Daddy. But regardless of whether it was convenient or not, there was no question as to what our action would be. We would welcome this child into the world and into our lives.

The remainder of the day was spent attempting to regain a sense of familiar routine, but it was to no avail. There were just too many things that felt different—the most predominant being the degree of seriousness we seemed to have suddenly acquired. We were sure that regardless of what was going to happen, the forces governing the universe would remain intact. Our uncertainty, however, lay in the matter of what roles we would each continue to play.

Later that night, I was comforted that my wife seemed to find slumber with relative ease. I was glad that, at least for the moment, whatever demons she may have been wrestling with in her mind had been defeated. I kept faith that mine would be, too. But on this particular evening, the demons reigned.

Lying there with my eyes open, I placed my palm on the abdomen of the woman sleeping soundly beside me. I wondered if I might feel the movement from the life which was gaining size and strength, harbored within her womb. I didn't. Yet there was a sensation that I realized just the same—a sensation that, in spite of the demons at hand, compelled me to whisper ever so softly in the dark, "Wow, we're going to have a baby."

- 3 -

Knowledge. It's all about knowledge. With knowledge there is understanding. With understanding there is reason. With reason there is hope. With hope there is happiness. It's all a very simple process of moving from one point to another—provided, of course, that you have the knowledge to know where you're going.

This was the official doctrine by which, as an adult, I was coming more and more to live. Did I believe I had the power to alter that which had already been predestined to occur? Absolutely not. I did believe, however, that with the proper knowledge, I could certainly sidestep an unpleasant situation or two.

Now as my wife entered her third month of pregnancy, I came to the sobering realization that I possessed absolutely no knowledge about anything having to do with becoming a father. I found this very disturbing for, while I often had ventured openly into areas unknown, I couldn't help but think that the potential for error in undertaking such a monumental challenge as parenthood was extremely high. I turned inward in search of some prior experience that would provide me with the confidence I was seeking.

Let's see, there was eighth grade algebra. That was hard. Nah. I had all the answers in the back of the book. Okay. What about high school Spanish? That was really tough! Nah. I cheated on every test. All right, I've got it. What about my job? I couldn't have gotten this far without having some real talent for overcoming obstacles. Nah. I'm in sales. I'm paid solely on my ability to bullshit.

On and on I reflected, seeking the one shred of evidence to make me believe that I was in any way capable of facing up to my impending responsibility of Daddy. I never found it. I did, however, come to a shocking, but nevertheless honest, conclusion, which I believed just might save me after all. It was this: for the first time in my life, I couldn't count on getting through a tough ordeal by simply *winging* it. I would need to gain a sense of certainty — a certainty that would only come through the effort I was willing to put forth to acquire an appropriate education. Hence I began my quest for knowledge.

In a different time and place, I might have been compelled to climb high upon a mountain and seek the words of the great "wise man." This was the scene I envisioned as I buckled myself into my car in preparation for my less strenuous journey to the nearest major shopping mall. The ancients would be proud, however, that although virtually all the knowledge known to mankind has been conveniently accumulated within the space of a franchise book store, the concept of the great wise man has remained intact—albeit his name is now Fred, and his title has been reduced to Customer Service Representative.

"Can I help you find something, sir?"

"Yes. I'm looking for information on first time parenthood."

Without hesitation, Fred informed me that I would find all the knowledge I was seeking on aisle 33 A. As I pushed by the more carefree individuals who, apparently, had come this day merely to admire the abundantly stocked section of magazines, I couldn't help but think, *that Fred, what an all knowing guy*.

I turned the appropriate corner and there they stood, shining like bright beacons on a moonless night. Their descriptive and forthright titles seemed to give them a chest out/chin up stature that made them resemble a group of well trained soldiers, ready for battle at a moment's notice. As I examined the individual members of each row, I believed myself to take on the appearance of a general, reviewing his troops and conveying pleasure as only, "Mmmm, good. Very good."

After pacing the aisle several times, I found myself drawn to a particular work that, in subtitle, proclaimed itself as *The Complete Guide for Expectant Parents*. Normally such a bold statement would illicit nothing more than a sense of skepticism on my part. However, the fact that I had no reference point from which to gauge the book's content, coupled with its sheer size and weight, seduced me into the much more trusting attitude of "this is exactly what I'm looking for." I made my purchase, turned back to thank Fred for his insightful direction, then—literally armed with my bag full of knowledge—immediately returned home.

As I settled into my favorite chair to absorb *The Complete Guide for Expectant Parents*, I was reveling in the fact that in the course of a single hour on a Saturday morning, I had procured an immense volume of information that would comfort and prepare me for the radical changes that would be occurring in my life. It was with a great zeal, therefore, that I devoted the next nine hours of my existence toward nothing more than reading that book. Upon completing the final page, however, I acknowledged that neither the energy nor the enthusiasm I possessed earlier had prevailed.

Now, to say that my efforts had completely been for naught would be a grave injustice. For indeed, I did learn a lot.

I learned all about proper nutrition and exercise. I learned all about the physical characteristics of a fetus during the different stages of its development. I even learned how to prepare an existing child for the arrival of a newborn into the household. All of this was information that I believed one day would add immense value to my life. For right now, however, it didn't mean squat.

Let me just say first that the priority I was placing on my own needs was totally selfish. Without question, the proper care and nurturing of our unborn child was a major concern to me. But in spite of the fact that our society was closing in on a new century, the reality that I was not the one *carrying the child* compelled me to maintain a very old fashioned thought of "you take care of the child before it's born, and I'll take care of it after." As a result of my chauvinistic and archaic thinking, therefore, I had the luxury of worrying about the more intangible and ambiguous aspects of the pregnancy, as well as parenthood in general.

The burning questions to which I needed answers all fell

under the category, TELL ME IT'S GOING TO BE OKAY. These included, but were not limited to:

tell me I won't faint in the delivery room,

tell me I won't have to take out a second mortgage to pay the doctor bills,

tell me I won't secretly begin to admire my neighbor's mini van,

tell me I won't begin to suddenly lose my hair,

tell me I won't have to dress up as "The Tin Man" on Halloween,

tell me I won't have to get a cat and ruin all my furniture,

tell me I won't fall down the stairs tripping over a roller skate,

tell me I won't pretend to respect my boss because junior needs braces,

tell me I won't be revered as "the head dork" by acne-faced adolescents,

tell me I won't be discovered dead in my office at the age of forty-two.

These and many more like them were the hypothetical dilemmas running rampant in my mind over the prospect of becoming a father. It was clear to me that in spite of my limited efforts of reading only one book, the chances of finding these particular topics discussed openly in any of the available literature on pregnancy and new parenthood was downright slim to none. Still, I remained devoted to pursuing my quest for knowledge. As such, instead of continuing to try to learn from books, I embarked on what seemed to be a more appropriate strategy: one-on-one discussions with those who possessed firsthand experience.

In committing myself to actually inquire into the life experiences of others, it was crucial that I keep two very important things in mind. First was my high degree of vulnerability. As susceptible as I was for input, the wrong input could definitely do more harm than good. Second, in spite of my eagerness, I needed to always consider the source. Soliciting advice from a man who sat alone eating out of a can every night because he believed his wife and children had been tying him down, did seem a bit pointless. So it wasn't just experience that counted. I needed someone who was credible as well. Enter Uncle Neil.

It was true that we were worlds apart in both our politics and personalities. Fifteen years my senior, Uncle Neil (who was actually my wife's uncle) represented to me, however, the epitome of just how much one was capable of achieving in the way of domestic tranquillity. Beyond the feat of remaining happily married to the same woman for more than twenty years, he was also accredited as being half of the parental team that raised two absolutely beautiful children, who—by today's standards—would be considered as nothing less than perfect. Although a quiet man not readily accustomed to handing out advice, Uncle Neil was more than agreeable to having me stop by for a chat.

Sitting there intently huddled at the kitchen table of Uncle Neil's home, I was renewed with the same sense of anticipation I had felt upon first opening *The Complete Guide for Expectant Parents*. There I was with a "master," so to speak—a man who had not only faced, but who had emerged victoriously from, the challenges that I now feared. I might add that he had done it at a much earlier age and with far fewer resources than I already possessed. Surely this man was capable of providing me with the knowledge I was seeking in order to conquer the great task of parenthood and all that it entailed.

Over the course of the next three hours, I patiently listened as Uncle Neil reflected on twenty years of life as a parent. Through it all, I couldn't help wonder if perhaps I was alone in my demand to know the unquestionable truth that one could fulfill his role as a family man and still maintain a degree of individuality. For above and beyond anything else, what I most wanted my uncle to say was, "Yes, Steve, it will be okay." But he never said that.

What he did say was that I'd only get back as much as I was willing to put in and that every day of being a parent would bring about a whole new set of challenges. As for there being any secrets to success, there were none that he stated. It was simply all a process of taking one day at a time and doing the best you knew how. In considering that he had more or less guessed his own way through parenthood, he advised, "If you're going to wish for anything, wish for luck." And that was really about all there was to it. End of story. He then went on to show me the various rankings for the latest line of mini vans he'd been admiring.

As I said farewell to my uncle that afternoon, I thought again about setting out in search of that mountain somewhere with the old soul sitting on top, patiently waiting for somebody to show up. But then I realized how clouded I'd allowed my judgment to become. I was so obsessed with the fear of losing my own identity, I had completely failed to notice how surrounded I really was by an endless stream of evidence and testimony, all attempting to tell me "it would be okay."

There was laughter and music and art and everything else of beauty that the countless number of fathers who had gone before me had created. There was no doubt that they had all felt some type of anxiety with respect to their impending parental responsibilities. Yet they continued to move forward—long after obtaining the title of "daddy"—to achieve new heights of accomplishment. Why did I think that it would be any different for me?

Another key element that I began to consider was that in spite of my fear of incurring a permanent responsibility in my life, it had never occurred to me to take any other course than to readily welcome my child and to love and care for that child with every ounce of energy that I possessed. This was the indisputable fact that I tended to keep forgetting, while assessing my ability to succeed in a somewhat over demanding and unpredictable world.

Yes, I would make mistakes. I was quite sure of that. As for having to *toe the line* to better ensure the welfare of my family, that went without saying. But when I considered the countless number of ideas and projects I'd already abandoned, I wondered if perhaps it would be my child who would prove to be the catalyst for an entire new wave of inspiration, enabling me to take forth one of those ideas or projects to completion.

And then again, perhaps it would be solely through the aspirations of my child that I would be remembered for having walked on this earth. Either way, it was suddenly apparent that there was sufficiently more cause to celebrate the expectant new life of my child, than to mourn and fear for the demise of my existing lifestyle.

And so it was with elation, not dismay, that—speeding my European sports sedan past a line of several less aerodynamic mini vans—I officially resigned my "quest for knowledge." Life would forevermore be a series of unknowns and speculations, centered upon my desire to always do the right thing. All the books and all the talks in the world couldn't change that. Nor could I expect to find success simply by adhering to their advice. As fatalistic as that may have seemed, the plain truth was that life had always been that way for me as long as I could remember. So in essence, there really was no impending great departure from that which had been established long ago.

It was of some comfort to my wife, I'm sure, that as I entered our own home that afternoon, I was smiling and humming the famous Brahms lullaby. It was of even greater comfort, I would venture, that as I took her to my arms and held her tight, I whispered in her ear:

"I'm going to be a daddy."

Her response, although blunt, seemed to appropriately sum it up: "No shit."

- 4 -

I've always admired the power of the human spirit—from the slaves of Egypt to those of the plantation owners of the South, from the gallantry of those who stood fast on frozen soil at Valley Forge to the horror of those who stood in silence within the jungles of Vietnam. It's all there to testify to the human spirit's ability to overcome even the most insurmountable adversities.

As inclined as I am to focus on that which is the most dramatic, however, my admiration does extend beyond the matters of wars and civil injustice. Routinely, millions of people each day are faced with their own more subtle, less publicized, tests of adversity—lack of money, lack of love, lack of self-acceptance. These are all legitimate issues of hardship—a hardship that, overcome, equally deserves to be applauded for showing the ability to endure.

Up until this point in my life, I had never been confronted, at least knowingly, with a test of my own human spirit. Moreover, I was rather content with that claim. For although I had always enjoyed rooting for the hero depicted on the silver screen, the idea of personally having to endure any type of atrocity was wholly unappealing, even if it did mean the chance for immortality via celluloid. It was apparent, however, that as my wife entered her fourth month of pregnancy, the great test I had managed to avoid for so long was, indeed, upon me. It was, as I came to call it, the *test of man versus hormones*.

In retrospect, I can see that my present ability to accept that which occurs to me without the benefit of rhyme or reason is substantially higher than it was before the test. At the time, however, I was convinced that the fundamental aspects of logic which I had grown up believing had completely disappeared from the face of the earth. While there are numerous examples I feel a compulsion to cite, for the dual purpose of brevity and profound impact, I shall tell the tale of only one: the tale of New Year's Eve.

I'll begin by confessing that I've never been particularly fond of *The Holidays*. From the week before Thanksgiving to the day after Christmas, I've always found myself to be in a bit of a blue funk. Without going into specifics, I will say that the cause of my melancholy mood does fit the standard diagnosis found in your basic psychology 101 textbook. But regardless of the severity of my seasonal depression year in and year out, there had always been an antidote that enabled me to revert to my more typical, unburdened self. It was the date of December 31st.

I am, you see, an eternal optimist. Not only is my glass never *half empty*, I'll do everything I can to show that it is never less than *overflowing*. To me, therefore, New Year's Eve represents far more than just a time of renewed spirit. It is the ultimate, once-a-year opportunity to legitimately put behind me all those prior, little incidents which fall under the category of *Shit Happens*. The catch, of course, is that shit must not happen on this particular day of days. But enough of my emotional insight. On with the telling of the tale.

As was becoming our tradition, my wife and I had opted to stay at home to welcome in the new year. Along with one other couple, we held a very small, but nevertheless elegant, dinner party. My wife, I should note, is a tremendous hostess.

Now on a scale of one to ten, I would rank the time that I was having as a twelve. Every facet of the evening, in my eyes, was absolutely picturesque. This included the food, the conversation and the company. But best of all, I was with the one I truly loved. To quote a phrase, "It just didn't get any better than this."

At the stroke of midnight, Dick Clark officially announced the New Year. We all clinked glasses and joined in a rendition of "Auld Lang Syne"—nothing out of the ordinary, something that a lot of other people were doing at that moment. Also like a lot of other people (I assume)—with the grand event of watching the giant apple descend Times Square having been completed—I was prepared to more romantically welcome in the New Year via personal intimacy. At any rate, this was part of our tradition. Conveniently enough, by 12:30 a.m. our guests had departed.

In our earlier courting days, my wife and I would have forsaken all else to immediately commence our passion. But we were married now and in a *family way*. Regardless of the mood, it seemed only appropriate that we attempt to observe a sense of decorum. As a gentlemanly gesture, therefore, I suggested to my wife that she go on ahead to get ready for bed while I stayed to clean up the kitchen. Of course I had no intention of doing anything more than splashing around a little water and turning off a few lights. By the time my wife had gotten under the covers, I was already in the bathroom preparing for bed myself.

In total, it had been fewer than fifteen minutes since we had collectively, and in our most genuine portrayal of a happily married couple ready to show their physical appreciation for each other, bid *adieu* to our friends. Of those fifteen minutes, there were approximately only ten in which my wife and I had actually been apart. Granted they were ten minutes of not having the benefit of knowing each other's specific thoughts and actions. Still, how much can really go wrong in the time it takes to go to the bathroom? Apparently a lot can go wrong if you throw a few raging hormones into the picture.

As I climbed into bed, there was no mistaking that something had become terribly amiss. The harder I tried to get a little closer, the more persistently my wife tried to get a little farther away. Perplexed at the drastic change in mood, I finally sat up and inquired, "Honey, is anything the matter?" The answer that followed brought the shocking realization that two and two no longer equaled four.

Earlier in the evening, a topic of conversation had been about weddings. Specifically, I had been asked whether, in the event our child was to be born a girl, and if and when the time ever came that she wanted a big wedding, would I be willing to pay for it. My response had been—and I do remember it clearly—that if our daughter were truly in love and a big wedding was crucial to her marital bliss, then certainly. If, on the other hand, a big wedding was important only for the sake of *putting on a show*, then definitely not.

When given, I had regarded my answer as somewhat ambivalent. It was, after all, a hypothetical situation posed many years into the future. At the moment, however, considering that a certain part of my anatomy could have functioned as a hammer, I found the entire discussion downright absurd. Unfortunately, this was not an opinion I chose to keep to myself. (I know, I know. But alas, I am a man; therefore, I am stupid.) Like a raging river, the tears began to flow.

I discerned, between the heaving sobs of my wife, that I was without doubt, *the cheapest man alive*. The fact that I could even question paying for our daughter's wedding, regardless of whether or not we ever had a daughter, was absolutely horrid. It was also expressed that any man who would place money before his own child's happiness was absolutely unfit to live with. And so came the command:

"Get out."

"What?"

"Get out of the room, now."

"But--"

"I said leave the room."

"But, Honey, don't you think--"

"Get the hell out of here NOW!"

As I pondered a line of reasoning which might calm the storm that was now fully upon us, there were two things that told me I could not possibly overcome the elements of this argument. Number one was the conviction in my wife's voice as she requested my immediate departure from her presence. Number two was the conviction in her right hand as it met my face. A blanket and pillow in hand, I prudently retreated for an evening alone on the living room sofa.

From the perspective of the longevity of our overall relationship—some nearly four years—I fully accepted that from time to time there would be occasions on which I would find myself in this exact position (i.e., sleeping on the couch).

Never in my wildest imagination, however, could I envision it happening on such a special day of the year—and with virtually no clue as to the reasons why! I was devastated to think that I and the woman I loved were under the same roof, yet were separated by an anger so intense that the very outcome of the relationship itself could be tainted forever.

I lay alone in the dark, wondering if perhaps the marriage really was over. It was true that I had not exercised the greatest degree of sensitivity. But I'd been tried and sentenced, not to mention assaulted and ousted, without so much as the opportunity to be heard—and on New Year's Eve, to boot! If ever there were an argument for mental cruelty, surely this was it.

I was saddened to think of what a tragic way the new year had begun. I was unaware of any prior year having started on such a sour note, and I seriously questioned if this were indeed a prelude of things to come. The aspects of parenthood, after all, were such an unknown. Perhaps personal disappointment was something to which I really did need to become accustomed. As I neared my deepest despair, however, I suddenly remembered something my wife's doctor had said to me several weeks earlier:

"Unquestioning emotional support," provided by me to my wife for the duration of the pregnancy, "was of the utmost importance."

All at once it hit me like a ton of bricks. What I had failed to realize at the time was that the good doctor was attempting to give me a tip. He was trying to warn me in advance that unexpected, volatile behavior on the part of my wife was possible, due to the drastic changes her body was undergoing. Of course I would have appreciated it much more had he simply said, "Your wife might act a little crazy once in a while, but don't worry, it's just the hormones talking." I suppose, however, that there are codes and ethics that prohibit such candor. At any rate, I vowed right then and there to pay closer attention to anything our doctor might say in the future.

I was overcome with relief as I realized that there was no sufficient cause to seek legal representation. It had not been the beautiful woman who lay sleeping in the room down the hall that had lashed out against me this evening. It was the unseen enemy from within, some terribly disturbed imbalance of hormones that had launched the vicious attack. It was purely speculative, but I was willing to bet that come the dawn's light, the equation of two plus two might again equal four.

And so it was that I began to regard the downturn in the evening's events as merely my fate, providing yet one more opportunity to view the great holiday movie classic, "It's a Wonderful Life." I couldn't say that this was a particularly bad fate, either. Although I would much rather have felt the comfort of my wife's arms around me, Frank Capra's masterpiece was indeed one of my favorite movies of all time. It seemed symbolic, considering what I'd just been through, to be watching once again as George Bailey learned that, in spite of his never-ending trail of past disappointments, the life he'd led had truly been paved with fortune.

I was humbled now to think how easily, this evening, I had overlooked the many blessings in my life. I was not a wealthy man, but I was far from the hardships of poverty that millions of others in the world endured. There was love in my life—an immense love that filled me with joy and hope and inspired me to believe in myself. And in the not too distant future, there would be a child, a living legacy to the great love that my wife and I shared for each other. No, there was no mistaking that mine truly was a wonderful life. But for all my blessings, I couldn't erase the fact that I lay there alone on New Year's Eve, watching some damned old movie.

It wasn't fair. Come the morning, I would acknowledge that neither my life, nor its meaning, had diminished from what had transpired as a result of the unchained hormones running rampant within the body of my wife. But for the moment, it just wasn't fair.

I had everything a man could ask for, and yet I felt as if I were the most deprived soul who had ever walked the face of the earth. Beyond all else that I had, what I needed was this night. And so, although I could feel that familiar, emotional welt building as George was proclaimed "the richest man in town," I couldn't help but to mutter back,

"Piss off, George!"

- 5 -

I was sixteen when I began shaving on a regular basis. That translates to my having looked into a mirror practically every morning for nearly the past twelve years of my life. For all of those episodes, however, in which I was required to closely examine that part of my body which conveyed the truest expression of my character and being, not once had I ever recognized anything beyond the obvious of my outward appearance. On one particular cold and dreary winter's morning, however, standing there poised with lather in one hand and a razor in the other, I saw for the first time something more than just my reflection.

Gone was the familiar, carefree stubbly face, burdened by little thought other than the immediate task at hand. In its place was a visage dominated by a pair of very troubled eyes. They were dark and deep and bore an intensity that seemed to blot out the remainder of their corresponding features. It was as if they contained some message of great importance, the understanding of which was crucial at this specific point in my life. But what? And why?

Upon awakening that morning, I had conducted my standard ritual of putting on coffee, lighting that first cigarette of the day, then meandering over to the calendar that was tacked up to the kitchen wall. As for the first two items, they pertained to habits that had been formed long ago; I dare say they could have been performed almost unconsciously. The calendar portion of the routine, however, had been established far more recently. It represented a daily tribute to the status of my wife's pregnancy.

The idea, you see, was to keep me chronologically informed about the development of our child. The "fetus calendar," as my wife called it, measured a period of forty-two weeks. This was to coincide with the anticipated length of time that the pregnancy would last. Although there had been nothing written within the allotted space for this particular day, the small square itself had been heavily outlined in red ink. The significance of the mark was that we had now come halfway.

I was somewhat elated, of course, to think that the journey we had set upon could be considered as much over as it was begun. Still, it was with some ambivalence that I made the appropriate X and proceeded to prepare for the day of work that lay ahead. By this point, I had come to revere myself as one completely at peace with the prospect of impending parenthood. Yet as I prepared to shave, presented with a view through the windows of my mind, it was anything but peace that the eyes in the mirror conveyed.

I found myself becoming genuinely annoyed. Mentally retracing my earlier steps brought me to the conclusion that psychologically, something had gone click when I noted that my wife was now twenty-one weeks pregnant. Why it had happened, I had no idea. Nor did I much care. My only thought was to escape the piercing set of eyes before me. I focused back upon the mirror and delivered what I hoped would be a shattering blow:

"Look pal, just back off. I'm perfectly fine with this whole thing. I know we've hit the halfway mark, but don't sweat it. I've got everything under control. Wills, life insurance, college fund—it's all been handled. So why don't you just turn around and go back to wherever it is you came from and leave me alone, okay?"

Nothing, not even a flinch. My grand soliloquy bounced off that mirror like a rubber ball on a hard pavement. If anything, the eyes appeared even more relentless. There seemed no alternative to resigning myself to listen to whatever it was they had come to say. Begrudgingly, I inquired, "Okay, then so what?"

Now as much as I'd like to portray that the eyes—which, indeed, were my own—actually spoke to me, allow me to stop for a moment to put things back in perspective.

The communication that was taking place that morning as shaving cream melted through my fingers was not audible. Nor, for that matter, could I actually hear words, per se, within my own mind. It was rather like a mystical experience—nothing that you'd want to repeat around a water cooler, but something you couldn't quite deny when staring deep into a mirror. At any rate, the message was crystal clear:

IT'S TIME TO ACKNOWLEDGE THE IMPORTANCE OF PHYSICAL HEALTH.

It was a fact that I held a very limited affinity for alcohol and absolutely none at all for drugs. These were my good points and, to me, evidence enough that regardless of whatever fine line I may have been walking, I was far from falling off any edge. But there was another side of the story to tell.

I smoked heavily, at times almost incessantly. I drank coffee to the point where three to four hours of sleep a night were more than enough to keep me going. I readily ingested anything that was sufficient to block a few arteries—provided, of course, that it tasted good. Needless to say, exercise was not considered an important part of my daily routine.

These were practices that I had deemed as acceptable in conducting my life. The inclination to change may very well have been something I'd have thought of eventually. But it was solely the pair of ominous eyes that brought the subject to mind now.

In twenty-one weeks or less, I was going to become a father. It had suddenly become apparent that as a provider for my child, the very essence of my role was to do everything I could to ensure that I'd be around for a long time in which to provide. Continuing to ignore the potential ramifications of my present ways did seem a bit contradictory in respect to fulfilling that goal. My *wake up call* had obviously come, and I simply could not ignore it, roll over, and go back to sleep. And so, standing there holding nothing more than a sticky remnant of the fluffy white mound that had filled my palm, I vowed to get healthy.

All at once, the eyes in the mirror grew soft and compassionate. I had given the response they had hoped for and, in turn, I was permitted to continue on with my day. How I was going to continue with my life, however, I wasn't so sure. But on with the story.

In spite of the laughter that emanated from my wife as I relayed to her the earlier morning events, I had the overwhelming sense that she, too, like the eyes in the mirror, was relieved to hear of my newfound interest in taking greater care of my physical health. As a loving gesture emblematic of the wedding vows she'd pledged some seventeen months prior, she assured me of her wholehearted assistance on all matters pertaining to my diet. She also announced that effective immediately, all consumption of coffee past 8:00 p.m. would be restricted to decaffeinated only. As she put it, "Sleep is something that most people find they enjoy. Try it. You might like it."

It was comforting to think that half the battle could be won simply with the aid and support of the woman I loved. The second half of the battle, however—the issue of smoking and exercise—was my sole responsibility, and it could be conquered only from the strength and desire within myself. It was a sobering thought, and one which compelled me to question my fundamental ability to change. Regardless of what I perceived that ability to be, however, I was determined to physically start a new life. It began with the search for the perfect workout.

Now considering that I couldn't even recall the last time that I had purposefully engaged in any type of physical exertion, I suppose that anything as simple as jogging, tennis, handball, or even walking, could have provided the basic exercise my body needed. But I was a man willing to make a commitment. And for the contemporary man, commitment was reinforced by only one thing—major purchase—hence, the *NordicTrack.*

The NordicTrack is a sophisticated cross-country ski machine designed for a complete upper and lower body workout. Not to be confused with those $49.95 cheap imitations, it is quite an elaborate device.

Besides separate tension controls for both the arms and legs, the NordicTrack has numerous elevation settings. It is equipped with a stopwatch and odometer and can even be ordered with a pulse meter (sorry, no cruise control). Although it weighs about fifty pounds, it is fully portable. Keep in mind, however, that it is a rather bulky item to tote.

I was quoted standard delivery time from the manufacturer to be anywhere from fourteen to twenty-one days. It seemed a reasonable period of time to wait for such a miracle of modern fitness technology. But considering my desire to honor the commitment I had made, the time frame was completely unacceptable to me. Fortunately, as with most modern miracles these days, the NordicTrack could be expedited for anyone willing to cover the cost of express freight. There was no question in my mind, as I authorized the additional charge to my credit card, that this was the only appropriate action I could take. In turn, I was guaranteed delivery within three days.

The day the big box arrived, I was like a little kid on Christmas morning. Enthusiastically, I tore through the cardboard and began assembly procedures. A series of curses, some skinned knuckles, and an hour later, it was whole. I briefly perused the operator's manual and climbed on board.

As my arms swung back and forth, fingers clenched firmly around the hand grips, I had a vision of a Greek god-like figure performing with ease and grace. Imagine my surprise, then, when I combined the movement of my arms and legs and went crashing face first into the elongated steel bar in front of me. With both ego and chin sufficiently bruised, I dismounted the machine and again picked up the operator's manual.

Not having much of a reference point at which to gauge my physical ability, I felt fortunate to find a statement by the manufacturer claiming that mastering the coordination required by the machine could take a "series of tries." In fact, there was even a toll-free help line to call for assistance in technique. But determination and perseverance were the only assistance I needed.

Within a week, I was swishing my way back to health. Each day I increased the intensity of my workout until I reached what I considered to be the adequate level of smelliness and sweatiness. With a proper exercise routine now underway, I turned my attention toward the final obstacle of my new-found goal for health. This was, of course, my daily habit of cigarettes.

It was January 29th. As I sat contemplating the white-wrapped, cylindrical object burning between my fingers, I couldn't shake the feeling that it had been more than a mere addiction that had kept me as a loyal contributor to the state of Virginia's prime export.

For the previous fifteen years—more than half of my entire life—I had smoked a quantity of cigarettes numbering well into the thousands. Regardless of the justifiable criticisms affiliated with that statistic, I had found pleasure in every puff taken. But I knew that continuing on with this habit simply because I liked it would be bringing a very irresponsible attitude into my pending parental responsibilities. Like it or not, there was no alternative. I would have to quit.

I picked February 6th as the official date on which I would join the ranks of ex-smokers everywhere. What was the significance of this day? It was my birthday.

Like the true Aquarian that I am, I made it a point to broadcast to absolutely everyone I knew my intentions to quit smoking. In fact—in the same manner as fellow Aquarian, Babe Ruth, who purposefully took two strikes before slugging a home run he had claimed he would hit—I managed to smoke a bit more with each passing day, as I came closer to the target date. The Babe, by the way, was also born on February 6th.

D-Day arrived. Prior to going to sleep the night before, I had made sure that no cigarettes remained in the house. I had also taken the day off from work to avoid any external influence of job related stress. Unbeknownst to me, however, for the purpose of providing the moral support she felt I might need, my wife had also decided to take the day off.

Now, from my writings in the previous chapters, one may sense a rather twisted plot about to unfold. All I can say is that the old adage of "Never add fuel to a burning fire" should always be respected as a sound safety tip.

My plan, honestly, had been to lie on the couch and watch television all day. Although it might not have seemed to be the most rewarding way in which to spend a birthday, I personally considered it a great treat. Other than my standard half-hour of

Financial News Network every morning, television was not a luxury I normally enjoyed. Besides, given my anticipation of severe nicotine withdrawal, I could think of nothing more appropriate to do than nothing at all.

So there I was at 9:00 a.m., comfortably tucked in on the couch, fireplace aglow in the background, and LEAVE IT TO BEAVER on the screen. In spite of the absence of my faithful pack of companions, I really was quite at peace. I had been awake for more than two hours and was becoming increasingly convinced that the world was not going to come to an end. And then my wife entered the room.

"You're not just going to lie around all day, are you?"

"Well, as a matter of fact, Sweetie, that's exactly what I thought I'd do."

"Oh."

"Is there a problem?"

"No, no. It's your birthday, and if you just want to waste it, then I suppose that's your right."

"Well, Sweetheart, what would you rather I did today?"

"I don't know. I thought maybe we could go out together and look for some things for the baby's room."

Now by this point, I had reached for the remote control to turn off the television. I had also abandoned my prone position and was sitting upright.

"Well, yeah. I guess we could go look for some baby stuff."

"No, no. I can tell that you're not really interested in having this baby, so why should you even bother?"

"What do you mean I'm not interested in having this baby? I'm thrilled about having this baby."

"No, you're not! You think I'm ruining your life by giving you even more responsibility to worry about. You'll accuse me of tying you down with a family and then you'll start to resent me. It's obvious how unhappy you are!"

If there was anything that was obvious to me at that moment, it was how badly I wanted a cigarette. I understood that the verbal lashing I was receiving had been brought on simply because I was there, and not because of anything in particular I had done. Still, I couldn't help thinking that this was certainly not the time for emotional confrontation.

At any rate, I did indeed accompany my wife, after consoling her first, of course, on a day-long journey to review items for our child's nursery. Although my desire to smoke intensified as the day wore on, being in public did seem to at least assure my safety. I should note, however, that on our return home, I went directly to bed.

The next morning I woke up in some sort of a thick fog. I couldn't tell if it was from the lack of nicotine coursing through my veins or the fact that I had just slept for thirteen hours. Either way, my life all of a sudden felt terribly different.

I drove to work thinking long and hard about the challenging road before me. I had made the choice to travel the particular path I was on. But was it the right choice? Common sense said that it was. But as I envisioned a continuous series of turbulent events over the next four months without so much as a single cigarette to calm my nerves, the question of maintaining my sanity posed serious doubts.

As I pulled into the office parking lot, I honestly wondered — between the Jekyl and Hyde transformations of my wife and the cunning of corporate salesmanship — if there had not been a conspiracy planned all along. For, lo and behold, on the west side of the building stood a gigantic new billboard that—I swear—had not been there two days earlier. The advertisement read, "CAMEL, SEVENTY-FIVE YEARS AND STILL SMOKING."

With my hands tightly gripping the wheel, I knew that I had reached my limit. Once more I asked myself the question, "To smoke or not to smoke?" But staring up at the billboard proved too much to bear. I heard myself say, "Fuck it," as I threw the car back in drive and sped off to the nearest 7-Eleven.

I was completely out of control. Jamming the car into "park" as it bounced off the concrete curb, I proceeded to roughhouse an elderly individual struggling with the weight of the front door. Bullying my way to the counter, with a squinted eye and demanding tone, I uttered one word:

"Cigarettes!"

The pair of young, frightened, female eyes looking back at me told me that I was creating a scene. But I didn't care. My very survival at that moment seemed dependent on the endless rows of neatly packaged nicotine that she possessed. I barked again:

"C'mon, c'mon! Cigarettes!"

The helpless victim trapped behind the counter managed to stammer back:

"What kind of cigarettes would you like?"

I paused for a moment and then remembered the life-like desert animal puffing away in pleasure:

"Camels. Gimme' a pack of Camels."

Amazingly enough, I managed to refrain from immediately opening my new found pack of friends. I suppose it might have been some type of subconscious effort not to give in to the addiction that I believed would someday come back to haunt me. But the more apparent truth was that I'd decided that if I was going to blow it, I was at least going to be comfortable while doing so. It was for that reason that I turned left instead of right upon returning to the office parking lot and headed into a neighboring cafe.

I waited patiently for a cup of coffee. Nothing went better with a cigarette than a cup of coffee. When it arrived, I picked up the small package before me and carefully removed the top portion of the cellophane and foil. I tapped out the first of what I anticipated would be several smoked at that table and lit up.

It was pure heaven. I wouldn't go so far as to say it was as good as sex, but there was a tingling sensation connected to each little cloud of smoke exhaled. When I finished, I routinely reached for another.

I lit a match and brought it up to the tip of the fresh Camel dangling from my mouth. Just as I was about to take the draw that would connect the two as one, however, I stopped. It occurred to me that I didn't necessarily want to have another cigarette. I was merely acting out of mechanical habit. My thoughts then became focused once again on the late, great

Sultan of Swat, Babe Ruth.

There was no denying that I had taken an all or nothing approach toward my endeavor to quit smoking. This was, after all, the way I envisioned *The Babe* would have done it. But although Babe Ruth would always be remembered as possibly the best for knocking the ball out of the park, there were many players who had gained fame for their equally—albeit less spectacular—consistent contributions to the game. In other words, just because I couldn't hit a home run didn't mean I couldn't try to get a base hit.

I decided right then and there that, at least for the moment, I was not going to quit smoking. I did, however, commit myself to making an ongoing attempt to drastically reduce the number of cigarettes that I consumed. The goal would remain for me to eventually quit altogether. But for right now, I was more concerned with mastering moderation than achieving total abstinence.

So what's the point? I mean, what do Babe Ruth, cigarettes, a sophisticated exercise machine, and accosting innocent convenience store clerks have to do with becoming a father? Well, the point is this:

There is a single moment in that nine-month and some odd-week period of time that the entire concept of becoming a parent really all sinks in. For the expectant mother, I would venture that it occurs very early, perhaps with the first wave of nausea. For the expectant father, however, I believe that it occurs on a much more subtle basis—and only at some significant juncture in the pregnancy. Regardless of when it does occur, I'm convinced that for an expectant dad, a brisk walk down *introspective lane* is completely unavoidable. (As for me, I happened to be standing in front of a mirror at the time.)

While the prospective dad is on this trip inside, it is more than likely that he will discover something in need of repair that is crucial to his parental success. It could be anything from the amount of money he makes to the last time he paid tribute to his particular religious faith. As for me, it was a complete reevaluation of practices pertaining to my physical well-being.

I'm not trying to negate the importance of whatever

surfaces. I think my own case speaks for itself. I came to the realization, however, that it is imperative to keep things in proper perspective. An individual working at a car wash one day is not going to aspire to be the head of General Motors the next, simply because a baby is on the way.

Life is going to change, this is true. But the process in which life is conducted will continue as before. Goals will be achieved as they always have been, through both planning and persistence. All the urgency in the world cannot change that process.

As for Babe Ruth, what can I say? The man was simply extraordinary. It is interesting to note, however, that beyond his ability to lead the league in the number of home runs, he was also known throughout his career for the number of times he was struck out — a trivial fact, to say the least, but knowing it sure made me feel better.

- 6 -

Once upon a time, there lived a happy-go-lucky young boy. One day while on his travels, he stopped to watch two birds that he had noticed in a tree.

One of the birds was moving wildly about—hopping, turning, hopping, turning—almost as if it were in a state of panic. The other bird, however, appeared quite calm. Except for an occasional stern chirp to the first bird, it hardly did or said anything at all. After a short time, the bird who had been hopping and turning flew swiftly out of the tree and landed on the ground below.

The young boy was frozen with amazement as he watched the bird quickly grasp a scrap of paper with its beak and carry it back to the awaiting bird in the tree. The boy continued to watch silently as the bird repeated its action with a small twig and then again with a fallen leaf. He wondered what the bird was up to. Why was it working so furiously to deliver objects back to the other bird in the tree? Compelled to find an answer, the young boy ran all the way home to seek the wisdom of his older sister.

After he had explained what he'd seen, the boy's sister let out a hearty laugh. She was quite taken with her younger brother's curiosity.

"Well, my little brother, the birds are building a nest."

The young boy looked confused.

"Oh," he responded. "Well, what's a nest?"

Once again, his sister let out a laugh. She could see that she would need to be more thorough in order to satisfy her younger brother's inquisitive mind.

"Well, my little brother, the nest is like a house. The birds are building it so they can have children and all live as a family, just as we all live here. Do you understand?"

The young boy squinted one eye and looked back at his sister.

"I guess so. But why does the one bird have to do all the work?"

It was now the older sister who looked confused. She put her finger to her cheek as she searched for an answer to her younger brother's question. Finally, she found one.

"Because, my little brother, that's just the way it is."

The young boy tilted back his head.

"Oh. I get it."

The young boy considered questioning her further about what he had seen the birds doing, but he knew that his sister had given him the single greatest answer that any elder could ever give. And so he politely thanked her and continued on with his travels.

Many years passed, and the young boy grew to become a young man. One day he fell in love with a beautiful woman, and the two of them became husband and wife. Together, they purchased a home in a magical place called *Suburbia*. Not too long after, the young man learned that he and his wife were going to be blessed with a child of their very own.

The young man was very pleased and excited that he was going to become a father, but his wife was undergoing many changes that he did not understand. He was told that he and his wife would receive their child within nine months. He waited patiently, but with each passing day he became more and more confused by his wife's actions. Then one day, after waiting nearly six months, he recalled his experience as a young boy watching the two birds building a nest and the talk with his older sister which had followed. Suddenly, everything seemed to make sense.

"Because, my little brother, that's just the way it is."

* * *

According to my statistics, month six was the official start of what those in the medical profession have termed "the nesting phase." Nonmedically put, this was the point in my wife's pregnancy in which an extreme priority was placed on creating the most suitable home environment possible to which we would introduce our child. It was also the point at which, like the bird, I found myself hopping and turning and working furiously to deliver objects and perform tasks for my awaiting spouse.

Before I am forever branded as a *sexist pig*, let me start by declaring, "Yes, it is my every intention to portray the events of my wife's *nesting* in the most humorous manner I can muster." This is, after all, my prerogative. It is not my desire, however, to negate or diminish a woman's right to feel however she wants to feel because of the new life growing within her. As my wife often pointed out, "You walk around for a while like a stuffed suitcase and see if you don't act a little peculiar from time to time." At any rate, with that disclaimer in place, I shall proceed.

The *nest* in question (i.e., our home) was a four-and-a-half-year-old, three-bedroom, two-bath, two-story house. Although of only average construction, it was in immaculate condition throughout. (At least this had been one of the reasons that compelled us to purchase the house a year earlier). On closer inspection by my now pregnant wife, however, it was deemed that several opportunities for the nest's enhancement existed. These included rebuilding the front porch, refinishing the backyard deck, replacing a bathroom floor, and repainting the entire inside of the house. Total estimated cost? Three thousand dollars.

While there were several adjectives that could have accurately described my financial station in life, *affluent* was certainly not one of them. Nevertheless, through the combination of education, work ethic, and downright dumb luck, I did enjoy what I myself would term an *adequate* financial lifestyle. Beyond the trappings of a house in the *'burbs*, complete with a *yuppie*mobile in the garage, this translated into the ability of my wife and me to partake in a modest one-week vacation twice a year.

As an aspiring young executive working diligently to ascend—not to mention sustain my position on—the corporate ladder, I found that a sixty-hour work week was more routine than unique. Although I admit that my efforts, for the most part, had always been duly recognized, it was the ability to get away from it all every six months that enabled me to keep on functioning as a well-oiled machine. As the hand of fate would have it, however, it was as we approached the planning phase of our next intended hiatus that I was presented with *the list* of home improvement projects.

Dilemmas, dilemmas. There were two to be acknowledged. Dilemma number one: even if I were readily willing to substitute my frivolous want of a vacation for a more practical purpose of home improvement, the estimated cost of my wife's proposed repairs to the nest doubled what was actually available to spend. Dilemma number two: even if the dollars were readily available to spend, how could I explain—in a tactful and sensitive manner to my wife—that the projects she proposed were far from necessary and more a product of a hormonally stimulated imagination?

(Remember New Year's Eve?)

I submerged myself in deep thought (for all of about ten minutes), before realizing that there was only one course of appropriate action to take: I would concede to my wife's wishes and dedicate all available resources to the enhancement of the family nest.

"Wussyhood?" Perhaps. But I had to think beyond that. What lay before me was an opportunity to prove to my wife that the concern and importance she placed on the well-being of our child was equally shared by me. In fact, in addressing the discrepancy between the dollars needed and the dollars on hand, I saw no alternative but to take on the task of repainting the house myself. (I did, after all, have a week off on my hands). And so with nobility in my heart and about as much technical expertise to fill a thimble, the only trip I found myself taking was that to the neighborhood lumber yard.

Given the fact that I was born and, for the most part, raised in a metropolitan urban environment, I can say that I possess an inherent excuse for not being particularly wise to the *handyman* ways of suburban life. The truth of the matter, however, is that some people, myself especially, just weren't made to play with power tools. That's okay, though. For these are the people, myself especially, who were meant to carry a checkbook.

There had, indeed, been a precedent set which fully documented my lack of mechanical prowess. It had come in the form of an unsuccessful attempt at installing a new towel bar. For anyone wondering just how unsuccessful my attempt could have been, I will say that not only did I fail to hang the towel bar, but I also produced a total of six very large, very noticeable, gaping holes in the bathroom wall. And yes, I did write a check to cover the damage. At this juncture, however, I had to place that episode behind me.

Standing before a man named Milt, I realized the importance of my mission. I wasn't just looking to slap up a few gallons of paint and call it a day. I had made a commitment to personally contribute my efforts, my sweat, my ache, to the betterment of the nest. My failure to be successful could forever result in a stigma against my abilities as a parent. Today it was painting the house. Tomorrow it would be assembling a tricycle. GOD knows what might lie ahead from there.

I was determined, regardless of the absolute fear coursing through my body, not to show anything less than total confidence in the task I was about to undertake. This took a particular amount of courage, considering that I was the only one there wearing loafers.

"Milt, I got a big project ahead of me. I'm painting a house. I need paint, brushes, rollers, tarps, the whole nine yards. Think you can set me up?" (Now that was strategy for you: put Milt on the defensive.)

"Well, I think we can do 'er. Interior or exterior?"

"Excuse me?"

"You painting the inside or the outside?" (Damn, he caught me off guard on that one.)

"Umm, interior. I need your standard type of white paint."

"All right, that'd be a latex. How about a color?" (I was ready for this one).

"White. I'm paintin' 'er white, Milt."

"Exactly what color white would that be?"

"Excuse me?"

"Well, you got your off-white, your egg shell white, your antique white, your pearl white, your bone white, your..."

Beyond that point, I can't really remember how many more shades of white that Milt proceeded to rattle off. All I knew was that I was definitely in over my head. I had no choice. It was time to come clean.

"Look Milt, I'm going to be perfectly honest with you. I don't have a single clue what I'm doing. Maybe we can take this all over again from the beginning?"

What transpired from then on I will always regard as the epitome of proof that by nature, man is good. There I was, a *city slicker*, completely out of my element. Rather than being treated with intolerance, however, upon regaling Milt and everyone else within earshot with the entire story of why I had to do what I had no idea how to do, I was befriended by all.

It was more than just kindly assistance that Milt and the others extended to me. It was an act of charitable consensus, one which consisted of in-depth swatch analysis, masking technique, putty procedures and, of course, the art of the *stroke* itself. I believe the highlight of the group's compassion, however, was displayed in a minor brawl which broke out over the question of whether *we* should go with the more traditional metal paint pan or the newly introduced plastic pan. As a sign of my respect and appreciation to all, I purchased one of each. In the end, I had been unanimously assured that I possessed everything I could possibly need to take on the task of repainting the nest.

As I hailed farewell to my new-found group of comrades, I couldn't help but feel that I was departing with a little bit of sense and spirit of each of them. I had entered that lumber yard as an outsider. However, through the commonalty of parenthood and the paternal notion to protect and provide a better way of life for those we have ourselves created, I had been accepted as one of their own. It was comforting to think that regardless of how incapable I really was to be left unsupervised with something as permanent as a can of paint, somewhere out there, somebody was cheering me on.

Now prior to my departure for supplies that morning, my wife had announced that she would be staying with some friends of ours for the next several days. I understood this, considering that the smell of paint is disturbing enough under normal conditions, let alone trying to endure it on top of being six months pregnant. Still, I was surprised after being gone only two hours to discover the speed with which she had vacated the premises. I found a note tacked to the door:

Steven, went to Jenn's. Let me know when it's safe to return.

Love A

So that's the way it was going to be, was it? Get out while the getting is good? Well, I really couldn't blame her. Given the opportunity, I would gladly have deserted myself. But that was fantasy.

The cold reality was that the fate of the nest lay on my shoulders, and my shoulders alone. It was up to me, Dad, to bring the ship safely back to port. According to Milt, I had all the *right stuff*. It was a question of whether I had the heart to keep on going. Surprisingly enough, it turned out that I did.

Four days later, I emerged, completely oblivious to the general events of the outside world, but intensely cognizant of the fact that I had succeeded with what I had specifically set out to do. All designated areas had been painted and—if I may add—not too shabbily so.

The sense of accomplishment that I felt over painting that house was absolutely unequaled by anything I had ever known before. I knew that in spite of my many years of white collar encapsulation, I had proven myself worthy to be matched *mano e mano* against the element of do-it-yourself suburbia. I could now consider myself a member of that elite group of individuals who could boldly say they had shown "pride of ownership."

Standing back reflecting on my efforts, I was compelled to think of the great patriot Francis Scott Key. As the smoke—er, I mean fumes—cleared, the nest (like the flag) had shown through the night. With all furnishings appropriately back in place, I telephoned my wife that a state of peace was once again at hand.

With the completion of my project, every item on my wife's original list of home improvement repairs had been satisfied. I deemed it a safe assumption, therefore, that all matters pertaining to the nest had been sufficiently squared away. Upon my wife's return, however, after perusing my work—to which she professed her utter amazement—she informed me that we were now set "to begin to get to work for the arrival of our child." My intelligent response to that remark was, "Huh?"

As my wife explained it, as important as it was that our home be spotless and structurally sound for the arrival of our child, it was equally important, if not more so, that we possess the necessary equipment within the home in order to administer the proper care to our child. Specifically, she was talking about our need to purchase a few items. These included, but were not limited to, the following: crib, portable crib, changing table, high chair, car seat, playpen, carrier, stroller, baby swing, baby gates, baby latches, baby monitor, diaper bag, diapers, bottles, disposable bottles, formula, etcetera, etcetera, etcetera.

In spite of my natural tendency to provoke confrontation, I knew better than to even think about opening my mouth on this one. I was willing to accept that all of the items my wife prescribed were indeed essential for the rearing of a child in modern times. What I could not accept, however, was the sense of urgency my wife was placing on obtaining these items. Our baby was, after all, not even due for another three months. I was resigned to realize, however—throughout my wife's nesting phase—a whole new meaning to the concept of priorities. Case in point: *The Rocking Chair Incident.*

Under the guidance of my wife, who showed all the determination and tracking sense of a big game hunter, we managed to virtually bag everything we were looking for in a little less than the course of two days. The majority of items were purchased at major department stores, so there was no real concern in transporting larger things home. There was one item, however—an oversized rocking chair—that my wife picked out from a specialty furniture store which, unfortunately, did not provide the service of home delivery.

In retrospect, I suppose it would have been a lot less

unnerving to simply rent a moving van to get that rocking chair from its place of origin to our baby's nursery. But since my wife assured me that she had a *connection* in the way of borrowing a friend's pickup truck, I was relatively at ease in assuming that that rocking chair would indeed find its way to our child's room. As with most of my assumptions during this particular period of time, however, I was dead wrong.

For some reason, my wife developed an acute case of shyness in approaching her friend for the use of the truck. Each morning I would leave for work, and each morning my wife would assure me that today she would call her friend to arrange for a time to pick up the chair. Each night upon my return, however, I would find my wife sulking and despondent on the living room couch.

"Honey, what's the matter?"

"You don't love me."

"Of course I love you."

"No, you don't. If you loved me, you'd get my rocking chair."

"Honey, you are getting your rocking chair. We're just waiting to borrow your friend's truck so we can pick it up. Remember?"

"No, you won't let me have my rocking chair. Our baby could come at any time and I won't be ready?"

"What do you mean, 'You won't be ready'?"

"I told you. I don't have a rocking chair. I'm not prepared to have a baby."

Now this was usually the point at which I would make the mistake of attempting to inject a shot of logic into the conversation. I knew it was futile and downright antagonizing, but my ignorance always seemed to prevail.

"First of all, the baby isn't even due for another three months, and second, what does a rocking chair have to do with having a baby anyway?"

"There, you see? YOU don't think I should have a rocking chair. YOU don't think it's important. Well, let me tell you something, mister. I don't need YOU to take care of me. I'll get a job and buy my own damn rocking chair!"

SLAM! BANG! CRASH!

The argument always climaxed with my wife's reeling herself off the couch and making a beeline for the suitcases in the garage. Of course I was always one step behind her apologizing profusely for being so insensitive and assuring her that the rocking chair would be hers once we could arrange to bring it home.

Fortunately for me, my wife never did actually pack, although there was more than one occasion when I thought she really would. When it had gotten to the point, however, that I was offering to help her pack, I knew that we had both had enough.

After a solid week of doing our best "Ralph and Alice" imitations, I personally phoned my wife's friend, whom I didn't know, and explained our situation. Less than twenty-four hours later, the prized chair occupied its intended space in the corner of our unborn child's room.

As my wife pressed down against the sturdy oak beneath her, she began to cry. I proceeded with caution as I asked, "Now what's wrong?"

Eyes closed, and in a little more than a whisper she answered, "I can finally relax."

"Why is that, Sweetheart?"

"I'm finally ready to have this baby."

At last, the nest was done.

- 7 -

As a kid, there was nothing I loved more than tagging along with my older brothers to see the Mets play baseball at Shea Stadium. Because there were five of us, there was always a consideration to be paid for our collective price of admission. The ticket I was handed was always for a seat way up high in a section simply known as *the bleachers*.

Regardless of my particular vantage point, it was always gratitude that I expressed to my older siblings for the opportunity just to be there. Still, I couldn't help being somewhat envious of those more financially fortunate seated down below, who, I believed, at least had a calculable chance of leaving that ball park with the one thing every eleven-year-old dreamed of: a retrieved foul ball. But then I saw something happen that made me think watching the game from the *cheap seats* really wasn't so bad after all.

One brilliant sunny afternoon, as the planes screamed overhead enroute to LaGuardia Airport, a line drive, resembling the flight of a little round rocket, was launched into the seats just above the third base dugout. While I could appreciate the magnanimous effort behind the spectator's outstretched hand, I could be heard (along with about fifty thousand others) to utter nothing more than "Ooooooo," as they extracted the unconscious man from his very expensive, phenomenally located, box seat.

From that day on, whenever my brothers and I returned to Shea Stadium, I never again questioned, nor cursed, the forces that limited me to observe the Mets from some perch high above. Although it was unlikely that I'd ever catch a foul ball from where I sat, I would most likely be protected from ever getting hit by one also. Hence I adopted the credo, "with distance comes safety."

Throughout the first six months of my wife's pregnancy, I had most certainly kept my distance. Noble or not, it was the only position in which I could find any comfort, and I dare say, it was the only position I intended to take until it was time for me to hand out cigars. Upon entering month seven, however, the notion I had of maintaining a safe distance for the duration of the pregnancy was completely obliterated by my wife, who insisted that I, like the unsuspecting fool whom I'd watched get *beaned* some sixteen years earlier, assume a new position directly in the line of fire. I'm speaking, of course, about childbirth classes.

I couldn't say that I had anything particularly against learning all about the miracle of birth. It was a fascinating process, I was sure—one which, if I could say I knew anything about it, might one day make for some really intelligent, fireside conversation. But the idea of my being present in the room and—as I'd heard the phrase used—*assisting with the delivery of the child* was enough to make me want to turn and head for the hills.

The problem, you see, was that for all the brash and bravado that I outwardly displayed, on a deeper level I possessed the constitution of a wet sponge. I mean it was troubling enough to have to deal with the *accident* the dog had left on the kitchen floor. But to watch a baby being born? C'mon! Nevertheless, the expectation by my wife was that for two hours every Thursday evening for the next eight weeks, I would willingly and cooperatively attend a childbirth class. The idea, as she put it, was to prepare me for my *instrumental contribution* toward the delivery of our child.

I suppose that to the highly trained, analytical professional, (a.k.a. *shrink*), the enormous anxiety I felt over the prospect of being up close and personal at the time of our child's arrival might simply be classified as a typical male *last chance to show some real fear of becoming a parent* reaction. And truthfully, I was afraid—but not because of becoming a parent.

The fear I had stemmed wholly from my belief that at the time of the big event, I would surely pass out, hence causing some major distraction to the medical staff, who were being paid (and quite handsomely, I might add) for doing their job, which was, of course, to deliver my child. Had I ever had the inclination to play doctor past the age of nine, I'd have gone to school and gotten a degree that said I was qualified to do so. The degree that I proudly displayed on my wall was for majoring in English, with an emphasis in literature. This does not an obstetrician make.

But these were the *nineties*, and the carefree days of the expectant father's being allowed to pace the halls with a doll in one hand and a football in the other were long gone. I was a victim of the enlightened man's theory of *paternal bonding*, which stated that a father's attachment to his child would be greatly enhanced if he were among the very first to help welcome the infant into its bold new world. I admit that it sounded plausible. But I couldn't imagine—even if I were able to actually remain on my feet during the great event—greeting my child in any other way, as it passed through its portal, than with my eyes tightly shut.

Again, I'll acknowledge that the way I anticipated I was going to react might easily have been dismissed—by one with the statistics to prove it—as nothing more than a typical paranoia. Unfortunately, this provided neither solace nor motivation for me. While I had always believed in statistics, I also had to judge myself on the irrefutable evidence attesting to my sensitive nature. Specifically, I'm speaking about the severe degree of sympathy pains I had already exhibited. Case in point: *The back incident.*

From the onset of the pregnancy, my wife and I had agreed that we would meet once a week for lunch. With all the changes that we envisioned our impending parental status would bring, we believed that it was crucial for us to make a consistent effort, to ensure that the closeness of our relationship as man and wife remain intact. By choice, we scheduled every fourth lunch date to coincide with the day of my wife's monthly visit to the doctor. These were always the most memorable dates, for beyond mere nourishment and companionship, they also provided a *news* report.

There was one particular occasion in which my wife was

relaying the doctor's prognosis and recommended treatment for recent back pains she'd been having. The fetus, at this point in its development, had turned toward the spine. Although this was conversation that compelled me to order nothing more than water, my wife went on to inform me that what she had been experiencing was considered normal, and there was no need for alarm. Furthermore, the only real prescribed cure was a daily massage to the tender area.

I must confess that by the time I had escorted my wife back to her car, I was completely devoid of any conscious thought regarding our child's position within her body. It wasn't that I lacked compassion for the situation. It was simply the case of my running behind for an extremely important meeting. I did, in fact, exit the parking lot like *a bat out of hell*, and with a bit of creative driving, I managed to make my appointment less than several minutes late.

Although I was somewhat ruffled from my hurried entrance, I considered myself quite prepared for the meeting and, as such, proceeded with confidence as I was ushered back to the prospective client's office. You can imagine my surprise, then, as I reached to accept the client's extended hand, that instead of the usual pleasantries of, "Hello, nice to meet you," what came out of my mouth was a blood curdling scream that was as one witness described, "capable of stopping a charging Rhino."

Without warning and for no apparent physical reason, my back had been transformed from a combination of blood, muscle and tissue into a burning bed of coals. I was literally paralyzed, and with the continuation of the audible signs of my discomfort, I was instantly surrounded by an audience of very nervous office staff. Ironically, by the time a consensus had been reached that I be placed on a nearby couch, the excruciating pain in my back had totally ceased. I professed my ability to continue with the meeting, but I was advised to seek "medical treatment." The symptoms never recurred.

But let's get back to the matter of the childbirth classes.

I had concluded that it was simply not possible for me to partake in the birthing of our child. I was sure to incur a tremendous wrath—both from society for my display of cowardice and from my wife for my ability to so irrevocably disappoint her—but there was nothing I could do. Regardless of anyone else's expectations, my decision was based on what I perceived as my own limitations. All that remained was for me to inform my wife and accept the consequences.

For two days I conducted countless conversations with myself. I was hoping to discover some magical way in which I could break the news without breaking my wife's heart in the process. I never found it. On top of everything else, it was now less than three days from the time of the first scheduled class. I decided that upon my return from work that night, I would simply have to *come out with it*.

A few hours later I found myself frozen on our front porch. I could hear my mind commanding: *Open the door, open the door.* But I couldn't move my arm. Then the door opened from the inside.

"I thought I heard somebody out here. Come on in. I've been dying to show you what I bought for birth class."

Contrary to my wife's vivacious step, my own gait portrayed something closer to a death march as I followed her down the hall. It was all of fifteen paces, but it felt like miles. When we reached the living room, there, in the middle of the floor, was a full size air mattress with matching pillows.

"Isn't it great? It'll be real comfortable for doing breathing exercises. And look! I got something for you, too."

From a bag obscured by the couch, my wife produced a bright red, designer sweat suit.

"To be a good coach, you'll need to be comfortable too."

It was unbearable. The word "coach," which was the term used to describe the father's participation in the birth, reverberated in my ears. I had to tell my wife the truth, and fast. "Honey, I need to tell you something about me going with you to birth class. I..."

Before I could continue, my wife quickly put her arms around me and gave me the kind of kiss that made me remember why I got married in the first place.

"I have something to tell you about birth class, also."

"Oh?" (I chose not to interrupt.)

"I just wanted to say thank you. I know how uncomfortable you are about this whole thing, and I really appreciate you going through with this. Just knowing you're there will be so reassuring. I honestly don't think that I could get through this without you. You're absolutely wonderful, and I love you."

(Once again, another great kiss.)

"Now what was it that you wanted to tell me?"

Whatever it was that I had planned to say about backing out at the last minute had magically disappeared, for the only words I could say as I stared deep into my wife's beautiful brown eyes were, "I'll be there."

To quote Ripley, "believe it or not," the quick change of mind about where I'd be at the time of our child's birth went far beyond an intention of merely pacifying my wife. The decision, I swear, was based solely on my wife's uncanny ability to put the whole situation back in perspective.

I realized in an instant that the importance of being by my wife's side as she delivered our child had nothing to do with theories or notions pertaining to paternal bonding. Nor did it have to do with the off chance that I would find any of it even remotely interesting or enjoyable. The bottom line was that my wife was petrified of what she herself would be enduring, and all she was really asking from me was that I serve as the familiar face during her own anticipated time of need. This was a role that, in spite of my squeamish nature, an immense love for my wife more than qualified me to play.

And so I did, that Thursday night, accompany my wife to embark on a crash course on childbirth. Whether or not my presence would prove to be an asset could only be determined at the time of the birth. The same could be said regarding any speculation about whether my physical position would be vertical or horizontal. All I knew, at this point, was that regardless of whatever was going to happen, I was going to be there for it to happen to.

All prior negativity aside, the new objective really was for me to be the best student—and eventually, coach—that I could be. It was just a bit of bad fate, I suppose, that within the first five minutes of the class I became involved in a confrontation with the instructor. Before I go on to give a particular account, however, let me first say a few words about the instructor, herself, and a few of the other class attendees.

Except for myself and one other individual named Larry—who swore emphatically that he had always believed his pencil to be "without lead"—the majority of the expectant fathers, although nervous, appeared well read on the subject of birth and pregnancy in general. At least this was my perception, based on overhearing some of the small talk prior to class in which views on the subject were being exchanged. I, on the other hand, when asked my opinion on Doctor So-and-so's study of birth taking place underwater, had to confess that I hadn't actually done any reading on the matter, however, I was writing a book myself chronicling my wife's pregnancy. This was a revelation that typically produced an ambivalent response of, "Oh, how quaint," or, "Excuse me, but I see that the pitchers of orange juice have been refilled."

In no way did I take the lack of endorsement toward my literary endeavors as disheartening. In the same manner that I had chosen not to read the countless sources of material published by the medical aficionados, I understood that my book, too, might remain unread (if indeed ever published), and at best, could be used to shore up the short leg under a couch. All and all, it seemed a very equitable situation. But I digress.

The instructor, although somewhat plain looking, with thick-lensed glasses, was a very perky individual. Simultaneously, she was both revered and disliked by the pregnant members of the class. She was revered for her credentials, which included not only twelve years as a registered nurse, but firsthand knowledge of having experienced childbirth herself three times. She was disliked, however, for having maintained her "girlish figure," in spite of her mother-of-three status. The whispered consensus among the pregnant members of the room was, "I bet she doesn't even have a single stretch mark." But again, I digress.

After a *round-the-horn* type introduction of name, occupation, and expectation from the members of the class, a question was posed to the male attendees in the room.

"Let me see a show of hands from all the men here tonight who have put on weight during their wife's pregnancy."

I was guessing that the significance of the question asked was little more than an attempt by the instructor to introduce a bit of humor to the otherwise rigid audience before her. Beyond my own appreciation for comedy, I myself was registering several pounds heavier since the onset of my wife's pregnancy. It was my belief as well, gauging from the look of some of the other fathers around me, that I was not alone in my weight gain.

I readily moved my right arm, fully expecting to be joined by a number of my peers, not only with a show of hands, but with a jovial laugh as well. What I found instead was that I was the lone wolf in the room.

As the instructor glanced around the room and took note that it was my hand alone that was raised, she commented that it was quite normal for men to gain weight as a result of the stress and anxiety they might undergo during their wife's pregnancy. She also went on to say how surprised she was to see only one individual out of so many who had put on weight. This was followed with the direct remark to me: "I guess you're the only one here who suffers from stress."

By the sound of near unanimous laughter in my ears, I was correct in my original assumption that the instructor was merely attempting to inject a bit of levity into the room. I couldn't help feeling somewhat defensive about her comment, however, given my initial reluctance to be present in the class in the first place. I was compelled to offer a rebuttal.

"Excuse me, but I think that attributing whatever weight gain I may have experienced solely to stress and anxiety is incredibly naive."

It was apparent from the immediate silence that ensued that the proverbial gauntlet had been dropped. All eyes became fixed on our leader, who was no doubt prepared to stand firm behind her credentials. Lowering her glasses to the tip of her nose, she peered forward, and with a rather challenging tone inquired, "Oh, is that so?"

Like a tennis match, all eyes quickly focused back to me.

"Well, yes, as a matter of fact. As far as I'm concerned, the only reason I've put on any weight is because of the countless number of midnight cheeseburger and French fry cravings my wife has had for the last seven months."

The instructor's glasses, now completely removed, had been transformed into a pointer.

"Well, perhaps you can explain what your wife's cravings for cheeseburgers and fries has to do with YOU gaining weight?"

This part was easy.

"She refused to eat unless I ate with her."

Once again, there was the wonderful sound of laughter. This time, however, I joined in. Undeniably, in my mind, I had definitely scored the winning point. As for jumping over the net, however, that was a different story.

The sharp jab from my wife's elbow to my rib cage clearly expressed that the only thing I had accomplished in my bout with the instructor was to establish myself before the class as a coach with severe reservations and dubious sincerity—not to mention pointing out what a supreme *smart-ass* I could be. It also served as a reminder that the gratitude she had expressed several days earlier over my agreeing to attend the class would only go so far. In short, I was being warned to shut up and behave. While I have never considered myself a particularly bright individual, I was smart enough to know that it truly was in my best interest to comply.

So it was that for the remainder of that night, as well as the next seven consecutive Thursday evenings, I merely sat there and winced quietly. How much I actually learned was certainly questionable, due to the amount of course material I obtained with my eyes closed. It was somewhat comforting to note, however, that even those who had not so much as flinched during the depiction of changes in the internal organs, did act a bit peculiar when it came time to watch the film on Caesarean birth. I myself opted to spend the entire time of the film in the bathroom.

By the conclusion of the final class, my wife was eight days away from the projected due date of our child. I could sense that the instructor was concerned over the level of preparedness with which I was graduating the course—and rightfully so, for I was as sure as ever that whatever task or procedure I was supposedly responsible for would never take place due to my being incapacitated at the appropriate time.

But in spite of the somewhat technical, albeit limited, training I'd received, it was never my intention to be termed as "medically capable." It was also my understanding, based on every account I'd ever seen portrayed, that regardless of how skilled the expectant father may believe himself to be, it is all rendered completely useless due to the lack of cooperation from the expectant mother.

I can appreciate the observation from those who would say that my entire perception of childbirth had been severely distorted from watching "too much TV." I would point out, however, that it is indeed art which imitates life, and not the other way around. With that in my mind, it was my contention that the delivering female's response to the surgically dressed male's instruction to "breathe" (while she was mercilessly being made to produce a product the size of a small watermelon) would be, "I don't want to breathe. I want to punish you for doing this to me!"

This was exactly how I anticipated things would be at the time of my child's birth. My legitimate purpose for being in the room, if any, would be to serve as a one-hundred-and-eighty-pound punching bag. Come the time of my wife's excruciating pain, I would be the human bullet on which she would be told to, "Bite down."

This was the message I attempted to convey to the instructor when asked to critique what we had gotten from the class. Whether or not this message provided her any comfort regarding my ability to perform, I shall never know, for I did adhere to her request that we maintain our anonymity. I did, however, leave a clue that would perhaps at least bring me to mind as the possible author. I signed off by saying:

"Sincerely submitted by the man who would most likely be bruised and unconscious during the entire affair."

- 8 -

On the very last day of my senior year of high school, I was caught for skipping class. Without going into detail, let me just say that I was not held in especially high esteem by the school's administration for my respect for their authority. Because of the skipping incident, I was informed at 2:45 p.m., Friday afternoon, the last day of high school forever, that it was uncertain whether I would graduate on the following Tuesday.

Now as a wage-earning adult some ten years older with ready access to a fairly competent attorney, I can look back upon the situation and realize that the sentence proposed to befit my crime was truly ludicrous. I mean, let's face it, if skipping class were just provocation to deny one's diploma, then three-quarters of the senior class would have to be denied as well. At the time, however, without the benefit of an attorney and still very much a product of innocence, I wasn't so sure.

I had been instructed to go home and spend the weekend contemplating my actions, and that is exactly what I did. No parties, no merriment, just me sitting alone in a deep despair, believing that my world was about to come to an end. My parents were more than a bit surprised at my subdued behavior, given the countless times I had protested my participation in the public school system for the last twelve years. Again, in retrospect, the fact that my parents were never even made aware of my crime or potential punishment should have been the clue that the faculty was merely attempting to *get even*.

I, of course, did graduate that following Tuesday, and four years later, graduated from college as well. So all and all, I can look back upon the experience and surmise that when forced to wait a situation out, things certainly can turn out better than you expect. Unfortunately, this was a premise that never came to mind as I desperately sat idle, awaiting my child's appearance in the world.

Let's talk about due dates for a moment, shall we?

Back in what was determined to be about the eighth week of my wife's pregnancy, we were told to expect our child on or around May 26th. Almost seven months later, however, our doctor revised the due date to June 10th.

I was perfectly calm when told to wait an additional two weeks for the birth of our child. After all, as much as technology will try to tell us otherwise, Mother Nature has always enjoyed the final say. By June 20th, however, any semblance of patience that I previously possessed was completely gone, and I found myself—for lack of a better phrase—*going nuts*.

Every day forward that our child chose not to be present became an eternity all in itself. I would lie awake at night and watch my wife's stomach do a tremendous impersonation of a turbulent sea and wonder, *What the hell is it doing in there? Enough already, get out here!* For all my demanding thoughts, however, the child seemed quite determined to remain within the confines of its mother's womb.

I turned toward my job to help relieve the anxiety of wondering when our child would be born, but it was a futile attempt at best. I would sit in my office staring at whatever was placed before me—or simply out the window—and wait for the phone to ring informing me that it was time to go the the hospital. The only variation to this routine was when I would call home myself, about every twenty minutes, and badger my wife with the incessant question, "Anything yet?"

Of course, there never was *anything yet*, and my wife's response always remained the same:

"No, there is nothing happening! I told you I will let you know the minute something does happen. But until then, STOP BOTHERING ME!"

Beyond the inability to concentrate, I had an equal—if not greater—problem in trying to distract myself at work, and that was the countless advice being provided to me by my two hundred and forty-nine co-workers.

"No baby yet, huh?"

"Nope, not yet."

"Say, how late is your wife anyway?"

"About two weeks, but the doctor says that everything's fine."

"Has your wife tried eating pancakes?"

"Excuse me?"

"You know, pancakes. Oh, sure. When my wife was pregnant, she sat down one morning to a big plate of pancakes and three hours later, our little Jimmy was born. I'm telling you, she swears by 'em."

I heard everything from pancakes to pork chops as a sworn-by prescription for labor inducement. As absurd as any of the recommendations might have seemed, however, I faithfully relayed each and every one of them to my wife. It wasn't that I believed any of them would actually work. It's just that it made a perfect excuse for me to call home one more time to inquire, "Anything yet?"

It was more than just advice regarding my wife's condition that my fellow employees saw fit to give. The constant perplexed look on my face, coupled with the accelerated speed of my most basic mannerisms of walking and talking, compelled my peers to address the matter of my own well-being also.

I was regaled with stories of meditation, poker, bowling, skydiving, long walks, short walks, running in place, breathing in, breathing out, not breathing. They were all offered as possible solutions to help me relax. The most thought provoking idea, however, came from a kindly woman in the word processing department, who happened to be the mother of two herself.

"You know, my husband was just like you the entire time I was pregnant with both my kids."

"Really?"

"Oh sure. He was forever running around like a chicken with it's head cut off worrying about everything. But I'll tell you, there was a sure fire cure that worked every time to calm him down."

"Really? What was it?"

"Sex."

"Excuse me?"

"You know, sex. My husband and I would have sex every time he was feeling stressed out, right up until the time our kids were born. I'm telling you, it worked like a charm."

"That's very interesting. I'll think about it."

And indeed, I did think about it. I thought that if my nine-month-plus pregnant wife and I could have sex at an International House of Pancakes, I'd be just fine. Of course, that thought was meant entirely as a joke, and that's exactly how it was expressed and taken when conveyed to my wife. For all my desire to keep things on a jovial keel, however, I am compelled to digress for a moment and speak seriously about the subject of sex and how it was affected throughout my wife's pregnancy.

I can sum it all up in three words: THERE WASN'T ANY!

Okay, so I'm lying. To say, "There wasn't any," is saying there was none at all. There was some, just not very much. Practically none, but definitely some. Nowhere near, however, "a whole hell of a lot."

Admittedly, I have never conducted one iota of research pertaining to the female's pattern of sexuality during pregnancy. This is a particular point of fact that automatically discredits me from claiming to possess any legitimate degree of insight on the matter. Nevertheless, I have come up with a theory that at least attempts to explain the reason I personally wasn't getting any—or I should say, nowhere near "a whole hell of a lot." It is respectively:

The more emotionally comfortable a woman is with her appearance prior to becoming pregnant, the more emotionally uncomfortable she will become with it after.

Without question, and certainly not for the mere benefit of this book, I have always considered my wife's beauty as nothing less than spectacular. While I would not go so far as to say this was the opinion she herself maintained, I will say that the act of viewing herself in the mirror never resulted in a bout of depression. With each additional pound gained, however, it seemed that an equal measure of belief in her own desirability was lost. In turn, my wife became increasingly disinterested when it came to the matter of having sex.

The absolute irony of the situation was that the further the pregnancy progressed, the more attracted to my wife I became. The reason was simple in that, with each passing day, I was more convinced that the growing life I had helped to create had been created within the one person who, herself, meant more than life to me. Call it happiness, confidence, self-assurance, or anything you'd like. The bottom line was that I was definitely turned on. But for all my sincerity and eloquence in attempting to express my feelings to my wife, I was never as convincing as that damn little red needle on the scale.

"Honey, I want you to know that I've never been more in love with you than I am right now. I think that you're the most beautiful woman in the world."

"No, I'm not. I'm fat!"

"Honey, you're not fat. You're pregnant."

"Big deal. What's the difference?"

"The difference is that you're not putting on weight because of a few too many Twinkies and beer. You're carrying our child in there. The baby is the one getting bigger, not you."

"Then why am I the one getting stretch marks?"

"Good night, dear."

Now, by going back to the testimony of the kindly woman in the word processing department (who had used sex to ease her husband's anxiety), there is proof that a couple can continue a healthy and abundant sex life through the duration of the woman's pregnancy. To those incredibly blessed individuals of the world, I salute you. But to those less fortunate (myself included), I call upon you to heed the fact that you are not alone; contrary to your feelings of despair, tomorrow surely is another day.

From the onset of this writing, it has never been my intention, either directly or indirectly, to provide advice to anyone regarding anything. But sex being such a universal subject of priority for the majority of men everywhere, I sincerely believe I would be remiss if I were not to at least offer some signpost of direction for those who have not yet made the journey or for those who are finding the journey too difficult to bear. As such, I impart the following:

BE KIND

The man must never forget that he is equally responsible for his wife's unwanted physical form. He must never stop complimenting her for her beauty, nor stop bestowing her with romantic gifts of flowers, perfume and jewelry (if this is what she is accustomed to). And most of all, the man must **NEVER** say anything complimentary about another woman.

BE UNDERSTANDING

The man must realize that his wife's lack of desire for sex is due to drastic changes in her life, and it should not be taken personally. It is a temporary issue within the marriage—granted, a long temporary issue—but it will be overcome. Siblings prove this fact.

BE CREATIVE

The man must strive to channel his sexual energy through a creative outlet. He must diligently work to disprove any notion that men are prone to practice infidelity during their wives' pregnancies. Go bowling, collect stamps, take up horticulture. As for me, I wrote a book.

All right then, enough said.

Before going off on a tangent about sex, I was relaying my thoughts regarding the heightened anxiety I was feeling because of our child's being late. I had explained that by June 20th—ten days after the revised due date—whatever remaining patience I had to sustain me to the big event was gone. Seven days later, it was June 27th, and still no baby.

Now, although I hadn't paid too much attention during the classes on childbirth, I was aware that a fetus could only survive for so long within the mother's womb. Our doctor advised us that up to this point the baby was in no danger, and that all we should do was continue to wait. He did say, however, that if the baby hadn't been born by July 10th, he'd personally go in after it and retrieve it for us via caesarean procedures. This was news that left me in an utter state of elation.

In the same manner that the date of June 10th had set me off in a panic, the *come hell or high water date* of July 10th had completely eased my mind. I was convinced that—for whatever unknown reason—our child was not going to initiate being born. I could count on the next two weeks, therefore, as an opportunity to regain some degree of mental balance in my life. All I had to do was keep busy.

Once again, I turned to my work. This time, however, I took out some insurance. That same afternoon, June 27th, I committed to myself and my superiors to undertake two major projects, both of which were needed for review within the next several days.

My determination was like that of an Olympic athlete. The confidence I held in my own abilities had never been greater. And as for my energy level, it was at an all-time high. When I left the office at about 9:30 p.m., I was certain that for at least one day I had accomplished my goal to constructively pass time.

I believe that I was literally *beaming* as I drove home that night. For the first time in a long time, I had been able to remain focused with a purpose. No counting dots on ceiling tiles. No self imposed interruptions of scanning the humorous captions on my FAR SIDE calendar (standard Christmas stocking issue). And absolutely no sense of urgency to phone home every twenty minutes to inquire, "Anything yet?"

It was around 10:00 p.m. when I finally walked through the doorway. My wife, although tired, had an undeniable look of peace on her face that told me I had made her day just a bit better by leaving her alone. We had a quick dinner of leftovers, accompanied by a brisk conversation rehashing the day's events, and we were both nestled in bed by 11:30.

In retrospect, there were three very distinct things I can remember about going to bed that night. First was that I had fallen asleep almost the instant my head hit the pillows. Second, I was in a very deep and tranquil sleep. And third, it was at precisely 2:13 a.m. that my wife woke me to say that the baby appeared to be on its way.

To describe my immediate reaction to the announcement my wife had made, I will once again compare myself to an Olympic athlete. This time, however, I shall name my specific event as the high jump, for this is what I appeared to be doing as I leaped out of bed.

"I'm up, I'm up! Don't panic! (My wife was actually quite calm.) How do you know that the baby is coming?"

"Well, I've been having contractions every twenty minutes since about midnight, and my water is leaking. I think you should go call the hospital."

So here it was, the moment of truth. Never mind that the baby had changed its mind about allowing me another two weeks to get my life in order. This was the time for rational action on my part, and I needed to abide by that fact as I stumbled to the kitchen to phone the hospital.

"Hello, this is Mr. Berger calling. You have a preregistered maternity patient by the name of Anita Berger, that's A-N-I-T-A-B-E-R-G-E-R. It appears that my wife has gone into labor. We'll be ready to leave in a few minutes and should arrive at the hospital by two forty-five. Would you please call our doctor and have him meet us there?" (I was absolutely stunned at how well that all came out.)

"All right, Mr. Berger, you're doing fine. But I need to ask you a few questions. Has your wife's water broken?"

"No, but she says it's leaking."

"What about her contractions? How far apart are they?"

"About every twenty minutes."

"All right, Mr. Berger, we're almost done. I need to know the duration and intensity of the contractions. How long are they lasting and is your wife able to talk while they are occurring?"

At this point, I was striving to remain patient as I called back to my wife, whom I could still hear groaning in the other room.

"Honey, how long are the contractions lasting?"

"I don't know, I think about twenty seconds or so."

"Can you still talk while they're happening?"

"Yeah."

"All right, Sweetheart, just try to relax."

I removed my hand from the mouthpiece and resumed my conversation with the hospital.

"Okay, the contractions are lasting about twenty seconds and she can still talk while they are occurring. Would you please call the doctor now?"

"Mr. Berger, it appears your wife is in what we call pre-labor. There really is no need for her to come into the hospital until the contractions are about five minutes apart and their duration is greater than forty-five seconds. I would suggest that you continue to monitor your wife's activity and call us when she is closer to full labor. It's not that we don't appreciate your sense of emergency, it's just that your wife really would be a lot more comfortable waiting at home than she would be at the hospital."

"I understand. Thank you."

I hung up the phone and realized that emotionally, I was numb. I had said, "I understand," but really, I didn't. All I wanted was for my child to be born and then for me to peacefully continue on with my life. Not only had I been told that our child had basically turned in a *false alarm*, but it was also my unpleasant task, as well, to inform my wife that she was going to have to lie around the house and continue to groan for a while. Life seemed so unfair sometimes.

I proceeded back to the bedroom like the doomed messenger about to be shot for delivering the unwelcome message. After all, besides whatever emotional discomfort my wife had to endure, she was now in physical pain as well. To my amazement, however, upon my relaying that it could conceivably be some time yet before we would be making our way to the hospital, the only apparent reaction my wife displayed was that of joy.

"Oh good. That means I'll have time to take a bath." (Of course I remained as solid as a rock.)

"WHAT?"

"I'm going to take a nice, long, hot bath. It could be days before I get another chance."

"You're going to take a bath, now?"

"Yes, but I need you to do me a big favor first."

"What's that?"

"I'm really starving. Would you fix me a peanut butter and jelly sandwich?"

I was completely dumbfounded. None of this was at all as I'd seen portrayed in the movies. Nobody was scurrying around searching for clean sheets and towels. Nobody was boiling hot water. The mother-to-be, far from praying she would be able to make it to the hospital on time, was leisurely soaking in the tub enjoying a peanut butter and jelly sandwich. I, on the other hand, sat in the garage chain-smoking, while furiously dictating notes to be couriered back to the office (so much for credibility with my boss). In spite of it all, however, things did progress.

Throughout the course of the next three hours, I kept a faithful watch over the activities of my wife's abdomen. By 6:00 a.m. the contractions were five minutes apart, lasting forty-five seconds and strong enough to interrupt my wife's ability, or at least desire, to speak.

Once again, I went to phone the hospital. This time, upon providing my updated status report, I was given the go-ahead to immediately bring my wife in. My reaction, although of pure delight, consisted of only one word: "Yes!" I marched back into the bedroom, my head held high like the hunter victorious in his mission to find food.

It was rather odd that with all I had to say, I simply stood there, silent, smiling at my wife. I was searching for the words that would befit the monumental moment at hand. Unfortunately, I searched too long, and my train of thought was interrupted by my wife's abruptly inquiring,

"Well, what did they say?"

I gave up and merely let it come out as,

"It's show time, boys and girls."

- 9 -

There is a universal principle in every science which is stated thus: "For every action, there is an equal and opposite reaction." I have never had a mind for science, but as my wife was being admitted into the hospital that Wednesday morning, 6:15 a.m., June 28th, I was preoccupied with that particular theory.

As surely as someone would die this day, so was a new life to be born. It wasn't likely that I would have known those who had left. But among those arriving would be my child.

It was an incredible thought and perhaps the only justification needed when I considered what was left of my battered nerves.

We completed the routine paperwork, which was minimal thanks to the modern technique of *pre-admissio*n, and were quickly escorted up to a birthing room on the third floor.

I was literally amazed at the place in which my wife had been scheduled to perform her delivery. Far from being the cold, stark, white room that I had expected, the room was quite large and resembled a hotel suite, with its table and chairs, expressionistic artwork and tastefully painted walls. Even the equipment located around the bed looked more like a home entertainment center than mere machinery designed to monitor one's vital signs.

Things were definitely looking up. We were at the hospital among qualified professionals, my wife was moaning louder than ever—indicating to me that the baby's arrival was getting closer—and the accommodations were more than adequate. All in all, I was feeling okay.

Within several minutes a nurse appeared to conduct an examination. I was really quite prepared to remain and provide any moral support I might be able to give. Modesty, however, compelled my wife to request my immediate departure from the room. Simultaneously I was charged with making a series of phone calls to the pre-selected group of friends and family who, in my wife's opinion, would be just a bit better off by knowing the status of our impending child. So list in hand and a pack of cigarettes hidden in my sock, I set out to perform my very first, semi-official paternal task.

Now to me, there's something about telling the same story over and over again that tends to diminish my sense of enthusiasm. For the first few calls, I was like the kid in the proverbial candy store.

"Yeah, we're at the hospital. No, she's fine. We're in room 305. I can't believe it's really happening. This is so incredible!"

By about the fifth or sixth call, however, I was definitely a bit more reserved.

"Yeah, well, we're at the hospital. She's moaning a lot, but she's fine. I suppose I'm excited. I'll be really happy when this whole damn thing is over."

Of course, I really was excited. And as I was making my way back up to my wife, I once again began to feel like that kid in the candy store. But I discovered that all the shelves were empty as I beheld my wife, fully dressed, looking somewhat forlorn—although not moaning so much—sitting all alone on the bed.

"What's going on? What happened to the nurse?"

"She said I may not have the baby today. I've only dilated a centimeter and a half."

(This was medical jargon related to the fact that a woman's birth canal must open to ten centimeters in order for the baby's head to safely pass through.)

"So are they telling you to go back home?"

"They don't know yet. They want me to walk around the hospital for an hour to see if it helps me dilate any further."

I should note that up until this point, my wife had really been one hell of a trooper. It was now 7:00 a.m. She had been awake since midnight in anticipation of becoming a mother, and now she was being told to, literally, take a walk. Of all the tears I had ever seen her cry, the ones which fell from her eyes now tugged at my heart the most.

"It's all right, Sweetheart. If walking might help, then that's what we'll do."

"But I don't want to take a walk."

"I know, Honey, but I'll help you. C'mon."

And so for the next hour, we strolled up one hall and down the next. The contractions seemed to intensify, and with every twinge of pain that they brought, my wife's spirits became renewed that this, indeed, was the day our child would be born. At 8:00 a.m. we returned to the room for another examination. This time, however, I was adamant about staying.

"But I'm embarrassed to have you here. Wouldn't you like to go out again and sneak another cigarette?"

"Forget it. As far as I'm concerned, we're in this together. I want to be with you the whole way."

"Okay, but just turn you head."

It really did surprise me how drastically my attitude had changed. Up until a few hours ago, I would gladly have opted to be anywhere else. But I learned that the love and concern I held for my wife was far greater than my feeling of insecurity about how I'd act during a crisis. I still believed that eventually I would probably pass out. But I was no longer afraid.

The results from the second examination were far more encouraging than the first. Our sojourn through the hospital halls had produced a full centimeter's worth of progress. In turn, the nurse was quick to change her earlier sense of doubt.

"Well, all right then, Mrs. Berger, you'd better put on this hospital gown. It looks like you're going to have a baby sometime today."

The words were like a cool drink to a parched throat. We were still far from being home, but at least we weren't being told to *go* home. Once again we were instructed to walk for an hour. This time, however, my wife viewed the task far more optimistically.

Upon our return at 9:00 a.m., we had made yet another full centimeter's worth of progress. The feeling was now that at the present rate, our child would be born sometime around 2:00 p.m.

The command to walk had been retracted, and my wife was now permitted to merely lie in bed and moan comfortably. She had also been hooked up to a fetal monitor—a device, sort of like a seismograph—to measure the intensity of her contractions.

At 9:05 a.m., the first measured contraction digitally displayed the number 13—which according to my wife, "felt like a strong one." She made the mistake, however, of inquiring how high the machine registered, to which the nurse promptly replied, "130." The look of terror on my wife's face was enough to end the perpetuation of life once and for all. As she lay there anticipating the pain that would come, I sensed her thinking that the entire concept of having babies appeared to be far overrated and that we simply had not been behaving rationally in our endeavor to add another being to the world's population.

As for me—the heartless beast responsible for her present condition—I was wondering, with the abundance of technology that existed, why it was that science had yet to invent the machine capable of simulating childbirth long beforehand. It disturbed me to think that the only way my wife would know how she'd do during the actual process was the hard way, which was, of course, to simply do it.

But we are, to say the least, a clever species. And our thinking demands that we supplement our lack of absolute know-how with a substantial dose of subjectivity.

With respect to childbirth, it is common to call upon those perceived as possessing infinite wisdom through prior experience, asking them to serve as testaments that despite the unknowns, everything will turn out just fine. For the particular role they play, we refer to them as technical consultants. During a more affectionate moment, however, we refer to such a particular person as Mom.

Since my wife's mother had passed away, it was by default that the technical consultant came from my side of the family—although my mother, having reared seven little rascals herself, most likely would have landed the job anyway.

At any rate, allow me to preface the next several pages by saying that I love and respect my mother dearly, and that I am truly thankful for the tremendous sacrifices she endured to provide me with a better way of life. On the other side of the scale, however, I must also confess that my mother does have a habit of being a bit trying at times. Case in point: *the appliance incident*.

Several months after purchasing our house, my wife and I had invited my mother for a visit. Since we were first-time homeowners as well as being newlyweds, we were naturally very proud of our humble abode. We were also eager to gain my mother's approval as well. We soon discovered, however, that my mother's opinion wasn't quite the priority we thought it would be.

On the first morning following my mother's arrival, my wife and I made a point of getting up early and preparing an elaborate breakfast for our most important guest. Our timing was perfect, for as my mother was making her way down the stairs, my wife and I were placing the last items of food onto the dining room table.

As my mother walked into the room and beheld the sight of the efforts in her honor, I was counting on nothing less than a completely positive reaction. She did, indeed, express her liking of the bounty before her. The compliment she paid, however, was greatly diminished, due to its being preceded by a rather biting analysis of our home's heating system.

"Hey kids, there's something wrong with your thermostat. I woke up this morning freezing. Sure enough, I put my hand over the vent and the damn thing was blowing cold air. You'd better have that thing checked."

Granted, it was the middle of February, and the winter in Seattle with its accompaniment of rain could seem colder than the dry Nevada winter my mother was used to. Nevertheless, I found enough merit in her concern to immediately check the setting on the thermostat.

I went into the hall and observed that the little red needle was proudly poised at seventy-six degrees. I then proceeded to place my hand over the nearest heating vent. Contrary to what my mother had said, I was satisfied that the air being blown was definitely more hot than cold. I found myself muttering as I made my way back to the dining room, "What the hell is she talking about?"

After relaying to my mother that everything seemed to be working "just fine," I resumed my attempt to eat breakfast. Her persistence on the issue, however, compelled me to drop my fork and offer a conciliatory reply.

"Well, Ma, the furnace is on a timer. Maybe for the first few minutes from the time it goes on, the air starts out being cold and then gradually warms up. What do you think of that?"

"I still think you should get the damn thing checked."

My wife, being highly skilled in the art of diplomacy, could sense that there was a potential situation about to develop. Acting quickly, she asked to be passed the cream. It was an incredible tactic on her part, given that the container was empty and my mother was instantly compelled to go into the kitchen for more. In turn, my wife worked to extinguish whatever flames of tension that might be mounting within me.

"Honey, I know she drives you crazy sometimes, but she is your mother. She's only going to be here for a few days. So try to be nice, okay?"

My wife was absolutely right. My mother did deserve my respect, regardless of what she might do or say to annoy me. I considered myself to be somewhat of a man of tolerance, and if the task before me was to remain calm for the next several days, this indeed I could do.

I took a deep breath and regained my composure. I was feeling confident that I would get through my mother's visit without a single incident. Then from somewhere within the furthest depths of the refrigerator, there came a voice.

"Hey, kids, this damn thing isn't working right. Everything in here is warm."

Now honestly—and God forgive me—my initial thought was to insert the remaining portion of my mother's exposed body into the refrigerator and close the door. Fortunately, my wife was there once again to intercede, this time with a hard stare and a determined enunciation of my name, "Steevennn."

"It's okay, Ma. Don't worry about it. Just come on back and finish your breakfast."

The voice resumed, gaining volume as it approached the table, accompanied by a pitcher of cream.

"I'm telling you that refrigerator isn't set right. Everything in there feels like it's room temperature."

Once again, I set down my fork.

"Well, you know Ma, it's interesting. A few months ago when the delivery man installed it, he calibrated the temperature for us. We've never had a problem with anything being warm in there before. But if you think there's a problem, maybe we should have him come back out and recheck it."

Of course I had no intention of calling anybody to check anything. I was merely attempting to humor my mother for the purpose of avoiding confrontation and to prevent me from saying something really stupid. After all, who wants to worry about rotting in hell for the rest of his life?

This was an approach that should have worked for days on end. However, my mother's uncanny ability to critique whatever she encountered continued to tick away like a planted bomb.

After breakfast I suggested that my mother go watch television while I did the dishes. My wife had left to take a shower. But I had sworn upon my own recognizance that I would be a good boy. It was an easy promise to make, especially when I had stopped to ask myself, *How much trouble could somebody cause just watching TV?* What I had failed to take into account, however, was that I had just offered my mother the opportunity to examine yet one more of our major household appliances.

"Hey, the damn color on this TV is all screwed up."

Even if my wife had been present, I'm convinced that I still would have lost control. I had been thoroughly provoked beyond the point of tolerance and to quote a phrase, "was mad as hell and wasn't going to take it anymore." I marched into the living room to find my mother stooped over the television, grasping at every knob and button she could find.

"Listen you! The entire time that I lived under your roof, I never messed with your stuff. All I'm asking is that you show the same type of respect for my property as I did for yours."

"But I'm just trying to fix it."

"No. You can't fix something that isn't broken. What you're doing is fucking with it, so knock it off!"

Okay. So I was going to rot in hell. But at least I wasn't going to be alone. I had six brothers and sisters out there who had been going through the same ordeal at least once a year, long before I ever became a homeowner.

At any rate, this was the *technical consultant* who would provide solace through wisdom during those final hours in which my wife and I were becoming parents.

For whatever reason, it was simply not within the grand design of things for our child to be in any type of hurry to be born. Despite the earlier signs of progress, it was now five and a half hours later, and we were still no closer to having a baby than we were at 9:00 a.m. Witnessing my wife's obvious discomfort—which was occurring several times a minute—was frustrating enough. But there were two additional issues which had cropped up as well.

First, it had been more than fourteen hours since my wife had gone into labor. As I recalled bits and pieces of my childbirth training, it struck me that my wife was going to need an abundance of strength to get through the delivery of our baby, and there was no telling how much longer that would take. To my eye, it appeared that she was already nearing a level of complete exhaustion.

Second, as the day wore on, the number of well wishing spectators had increased dramatically. At one point I looked up to find that there were no fewer than a dozen non-medical people milling about the room, all waiting for something to happen. For their show of concern, I was genuinely touched. For the growing number of distractions they were injecting onto the scene, however, I was beginning to get more than a little pissed.

Beyond the incessant pacing, there was a constant stream of telephone calls, both incoming and outgoing. My mother was busy planning my next seven days worth of meals, which included inquiries regarding the inventory of my kitchen pantry. And I was receiving an offer, at least every fifteen minutes, to be relieved from assisting my wife with her breathing. The final straw, however, was when an argument ensued over which kind of pizza the gang should have delivered.

I had definitely had enough. The day was getting longer, and we were getting nowhere. Like it or not, the circumstances required that I assume a role of leadership and take immediate control of the situation at hand. I temporarily delegated my duties as coach, and left the room for a private consultation with the nurse in charge.

"Look, I'm not going to pretend that I know what I'm doing. But it seems to me that my wife can't take much more of this. Isn't there anything we can do to help her along?"

It was almost comical the way the nurse cupped her chin in her hand and stroked her cheek with her index finger.

"Hmm. Well, the next step would be to induce a higher stage of labor. We could do that by giving your wife Pitocin®. Let me call the doctor and see what he thinks."

We had both begun to turn when I suddenly remembered my problem number two.

"Oh, by the way, when you come back, I'd really appreciate it if you could get everyone the hell out of there. Tactfully, of course."

The nurse glanced back at the crowded room and smiled.

"I understand. I'll go ahead and post a no visitors sign."

As I watched the nurse go down the corridor, I was somewhat amazed that all it seemed to take was for me to speak up. Upon calling my little conference, I had half expected to be told to "shut up and sit down." It was flattering to think that I had some input into the matter, regardless of my qualifications, or lack thereof, behind which it was offered.

Now, speaking of qualifications, there is a very good reason why I have not bothered—up until this point—to devote any time to depicting the doctor chosen to deliver our child: he wasn't there. Allow me to digress from the events unfolding back in Birthing Room number 305 and provide a brief account on the matter of the missing doctor.

The era of the Communications Revolution, in many ways, has provided the ability to keep in touch while keeping out of sight. In turn, this has directly enhanced the level of efficiency at which the majority of jobs are performed these days. The individual who delivers babies for a living is certainly no exception.

To make a long story short, back in about the sixth month of my wife's pregnancy, I went to work for a peer company. We were fortunate in that my new employer was willing to assume medical coverage where my old company had stopped. Unfortunately, under the preferred health plan, my new employer did not recognize our choice of hospital, which was, of course, where our doctor conducted his practice. Ironically, however, although the new health plan did not recognize our choice of hospital, they did recognize our choice of doctor. (Go figure.)

At any rate, we changed hospitals but kept doctors. It was a convoluted mess, to say the least. But it was doable, so we did it. The consolation of it all—other than money—was that at worst, with traffic, our doctor was only twenty minutes away.

Upon placing my second call to the hospital some nine hours earlier, I had been given the green light to come on in with my wife. It was my expectation that, at the same time, our doctor was being told to come on in also. I considered this a reasonable expectation, given my belief that my wife was about to have a baby. I was quick to learn, however, that those possessing a greater experience in the matter did not share my same sense of urgency.

Because my wife had been diagnosed as being in such a low stage of labor, I was told that as yet, there was no real need for our doctor to be present. Of course it would have been nice to have the doctor there anyway, if for no other reason than to assure us that it was perfectly normal for my wife (who, keep in mind, had been at this since midnight some fifteen hours before) to only be *sort of* having a baby.

Nevertheless, our doctor, although physically absent, was

by our side the entire time electronically. Beyond the more conventional means of telephone communication, he was being kept apprised of my wife's status via computer screens and fax machines. Technically speaking, therefore, we really were receiving the best of care—provided, of course, that the power didn't go out.

The nurse did, indeed, make a call recommending that Pitocin® be administered to enhance my wife's labor. The doctor must have concurred, for a little after 3:00 p.m., my wife was given the stimulant to help speed things along. From this point on—and, I should add, all at once—the situation within Birthing Room 305 became increasingly intense.

My request to have all nonessential personnel removed had been honored. The only players now remaining were my wife, myself, and a substitute nurse—who, I assumed, was somewhat like the relief pitcher called in during the late innings to pick up the save.

The fetal monitor had previously been registering contractions around the mid to high twenties. Within moments, however, the digital display had jumped to the mid to high seventies, and was continuing to climb. In my job as coach, I was fortunate to have the monitor to alert me at the precise moment that a contraction was beginning to occur. In turn, I was able to actually prepare my wife for the impending shock. Although my informing her that she was about to feel pain didn't necessarily give me the impression that her pain was being diminished, I remained faithful in my task.

By 5:30 p.m., the contractions had broken through the confines of double digits. Coupled with the heightened degree of my wife's moaning, the nurse was compelled to offer a renewed sense of optimism that a child seemed to be attempting to be born. She announced that—subject to one last examination, "just to make sure"—it appeared to be time to summon the doctor.

In spite of its being only a speculative observation, I was inclined to agree with the nurse that the arduous wait appeared to be coming to a close. It had been longer than eleven hours since we had first occupied the room, and I couldn't imagine the present state of things continuing much longer. In the event that they could, however, I decided to take advantage of the temporary lull in action and quickly proceeded down to the parking lot to enjoy one last cigarette as a childless man.

In total, I had been gone from the room for less than ten minutes. The primary object of my absence, true, was to grab a quick smoke. Standing there alone, however, puffing away while gazing at the summer's setting sky, I was still hoping to magically discover the profound new credo which would facilitate my transition to parenthood. But alas, it never came.

I did walk away with one realization, though—there are times, particularly in situations like this, that there isn't a whole lot more to do than merely roll with the punches. That thought wasn't exactly the foundation for world peace, but given the news when I returned that my wife had made absolutely no progress in dilation—despite our efforts to assist with the Pitocin®—it seemed more than appropriate.

Without any medical basis to go on, I was of the mind that our child's birth by vaginal delivery was completely far fetched. The idea of continuing to wait for one part of my wife's anatomy to catch up with the actions of another seemed downright absurd, especially when I considered the immense pain my wife would be made to endure in the process. Qualified to do so or not, I offered an opinion that we *bag the breathing* and immediately establish Caesarean birth procedures.

Judging by the nurse's look of empathy, I got the distinct impression that I was not the only one who believed it was time for an alternative plan. She informed me, however, that during my brief hiatus to the parking lot, a call to the doctor had relayed an opposing opinion that a vaginal birth was still probable. Our instruction was to *keep on trying*. I had nothing but the highest respect for the doctor's integrity in trying to avoid a potentially undue surgery. Glancing down at the spent form of the one who now only slightly resembled the woman I knew and loved, however, I thought he was completely insane.

There was one consolation that he did offer, however. He authorized the nurse, upon her discretion and my consent, to administer my wife with the drug Stadol®.

Based on what I knew—which, granted, wasn't much—Stadol® was a relaxant that was sometimes used in the situation of a long and painful labor. Although it had a history of being very effective, it was also considered to be an extremely potent drug. The dilemma, therefore, was that—as research continues to show—drugs of almost any type administered during the latter stages of labor can pose a potential threat to the unborn child.

There was no question that I had to consider the possibility of something's going wrong. Causing harm to our child with a decision I had made—I knew—was a crime for which I would never be able to forgive myself. But as much as I had to think of the welfare of my child, I was consumed first and foremost with the welfare of my wife. Closing my eyes, I gave my consent for the drug to be administered.

Now, in all honesty, I've painted a picture that's somewhat distorted. It wasn't as if my wife were clinging onto life by a thread or anything. I'm simply of the belief that even the most evil person should be made to undergo only so much torture. At any rate, the Stadol® worked.

Witnessing the drug's rapid effect was fascinating. Within a minute my wife had relaxed to the point that she was actually sleeping right through the contractions. Whether or not her newly acquired state of comfort would be instrumental in achieving a sufficient dilation, I had no idea. I did know for a fact, however, that my decision to administer *the juice* had definitely eased her pain.

Once again we pressed on. The unspoken plan, however, seemed to be that we were only going to continue for as long as the Stadol® remained in effect, which in our case was about an hour and a half. It was after yet one more examination, about 7:00 p.m.—nearly thirteen hours since our arrival at the hospital and a total of nineteen since my wife had begun her labor the night before—that the nurse openly denounced any notion of our child's being born the way nature had intended.

"I think it's time that the doctor came in."

As I registered the nurse's words, I was fighting to keep my anger at bay, for after all, she had been merely following the doctor's orders as we persisted in dragging my wife through hell for the last several hours. I did, indeed, have a desire to punch out the good doctor when it was all said and done. But then I remembered the portion of the medical expense my insurance wasn't going to cover, and I realized that time served would only add insult to the already throbbing injury. So I simply smiled and said, "I'd really appreciate that. Thank you."

It was approximately 7:30 p.m. when the doctor arrived. It took all of about two minutes for him to poetically assess the situation as my wife's being *too small* and our child's being *too big* for a vaginal delivery. Consequently, he announced that there was no alternative than to proceed with a Caesarean birth.

More than ever, I was compelled to protest the doctor's reluctance to have made this determination sooner. The plain truth, however, was that I was grateful simply for the fact that he was there. I had to admit, as well, that as I watched him orchestrate the countless details in such a sure and expeditious manner, any question I had regarding his competency was more than answered.

As the preparations continued, it occurred to me that the gathering of our friends and family, still patiently awaiting the outcome of their long vigil, had absolutely no idea of what was about to take place. There was always the option of having someone sent to deliver a message. But the unwavering support that these people had shown, first throughout the day and now into the night, warranted far more than just a message from a stranger. I viewed it as my personal duty to provide the group with an update of sorts and hurriedly made my way to the visitor's lounge.

Standing there speechless before the audience of familiar faces, there was no denying the state of my own fatigue. The broken voice through which my words finally did manage to come was evidence, as well, of the fear I was fighting to suppress. But as tired and as scared as I was, among the people in that room I found an inspiration that, I knew, was going to enable me to stay strong.

If they had any questions, they never asked them. If they were worried, they never let it be seen. They seemed solely intent on conveying nothing beyond their well wishes and compassionate thoughts. Without its ever being said, I knew that whatever might happen I could always count on them to be there. It was probably the first time in my life that I really understood what being part of a family was all about.

I made it back to my wife just as she was being transferred from her bed to the mobile gurney. Continuing on to surgery, I kept thinking of my initial hesitation about being anywhere near the scene of our child's birth, let alone being present as my wife went under *the knife*. It seemed ironic to me now, since I couldn't even imagine the possibility of being anywhere else.

At exactly 8:37 p.m., I became a father. Our child was nine pounds, two and a half ounces, twenty-one inches long, with ten fingers, ten toes, and an innocence that pronounced all to be right in the world. I marveled at the absolute miracle of life as I reached out to be handed our child.

With a pounding heart and tear-filled eyes, I cradled the wrapped bundle tightly in my arms. It was a humbling experience, yet it never felt so good to be so humbled. I knew that my wife, although unable to hold the baby, shared my elation. I bowed to where she could see our child and gently kissed her lips.

"I love you, Mommy."

"I love you too, Daddy."

It had been the longest and happiest day of our lives. As much as we were both ready to call it a night, however, there was still the task remaining of introducing our child to those waiting on the floor above. We were severely taxed, emotionally as well as physically. Nevertheless, we were unwilling to end the event without a dramatic close.

Upon our child's birth, our guests had been informed that the surgery was indeed a success, and that both mother and child were doing well. As for the particulars of name and sex, however, we instructed that those details remain unknown until such time as given by the proud, new parents.

We returned to my wife's room and prepared for our child's debut. After settling my wife and allowing her time to marvel at the life she had produced, we summoned the nurse to ask that she retrieve our friends and family. The nurse was a kind-natured soul who willingly played the part of our accomplice. She re-entered the room, keeping the crowd at bay behind her, and announced, "Mr. & Mrs. Berger would like you all to meet..," to which I proudly turned and responded, "...our daughter, Ashley Elizabeth."

Epilogue

There you have it—chapter and verse, so to speak, of my journey to parenthood. Am I of the opinion that I've penned the definitive manifesto for expectant fathers everywhere? Hardly. Yet I'm determined to stand behind the merits of this book just the same.

It was never my intent to formally produce a product for publication. Quite the contrary. My initial literary objective was nothing more than that of release—a diary of sorts to assist me in coping with the immense anxiety I felt over my impending parental status.

At the time, I honestly believed that everything I was jotting down was wholly unique to me and my situation. When it was all said and done, however, I came to the conclusion that everything that had happened to me had surely happened to someone, somewhere, before. The burning question I began to ask, therefore, was, "Why didn't anybody ever bother to talk about it?"

So I found myself returning to the pages upon pages of my handwritten scrawl and, as evidenced by the neatly printed words before you, made the decision to go forth and make public some of the most personal details of my life (not to mention those of my poor, unsuspecting spouse).

But enough about motive. A word or two about content.

As an author, I accept the risk of public reproach. Let's face it—everyone's a critic. And rightfully so. But as I've stressed all along, the views I've presented are offered as nothing more than my own subjective opinion. So for anyone whose ire I've raised, PLEASE LET IT DOWN! I'll gladly concede to the possibility that I'm wrong and you're right. Okay? Okay.

All concessions aside, however, artistically speaking, I'm not a man completely without a cause. There is one issue regarding the content of this book on which I will defend myself to the very grave. That is the issue of truth.

Regardless of whatever "personal slant" I may have interjected, the account I've given of my wife's pregnancy and its surrounding events is, for the most part, exactly the way it happened. Granted, I've exercised a bit of poetic license here and there. But I assure you that the pertinent details portrayed are indeed fact and not fiction. What makes me so certain? Simple. I was taking notes.

The truth alone, however, shall not set me free, for what is truth without understanding? There needs to be a semblance of sense, as well, before I can say that I've expressed anything of value. Permit me then, via these final paragraphs, to attempt to bring forth *the meaning of it all*.

In the late nineteenth century, a man by the name of Charles Darwin published a work detailing his study on the birds of the Galapogos Islands. It was within this particular work that Darwin posed an argument that would influence whole societies for generations to come. So profound, in fact, was this argument that it became, in itself, a type of credo that was touted by presidents, kings, and captains of industry alike. I'm speaking, of course, of Darwin's thesis about *survival of the fittest*.

Now, for all its effect, what's interesting to note is that *survival of the fittest* is perhaps one of the most misunderstood ideas of all time. Contrary to common belief, Darwin wasn't referring to absolute strength as the key to survival. He was talking about adaptation—the ability to successfully conform to a changing environment. In a nutshell, the bending willow will weather the storm far better than the sturdy oak. Thus I give you *the meaning of it all*.

You see, the real conflict I faced in becoming a father was my struggle to conform to the monumental change that was about to take place in my life. My wants, my desires, my attitudes—all were being challenged. I was determined as hell to resist it every step of the way. But the more I continued to reflect on the various aspects of my life, the more I realized just how conforming I could be (hence my opening dissertation on *Rastus the Dachshund Dog*).

As I revel now in the growth of my child, I'm amazed that

I could ever have had anything but overwhelming thoughts of joy with which to occupy my mind, for joy is what she has truly brought me. As for everything else, I think John Lennon said it best: "Life is what happens to you while you're busy making other plans."